D0871930

DATE DUE

OCT 21 '96			
08			

The
Price
of a
Life

The Price of a Life

One Woman's Death from
Toxic Shock

TOM RILEY

ADLER&ADLER

Published by Adler & Adler, Publishers, Inc.
4550 Montgomery Avenue
Bethesda, Maryland 20814

Library of Congress Cataloging-in-Publication Data
Riley, Tom, 1929–
The price of a life.
1. Kehm, Mike—Trials, litigation, etc. 2. Procter &
Gamble Company—Trials, litigation, etc. 3. Products
liability—Medical instruments and apparatus—United
States. 4. Kehm, Patricia, d. 1980. 5. Tampons—
Complications and sequelae—United States. 6. Toxic
shock syndrome—United States. I. Title.
KF228.K44R55   1986   346.7303'82'0269   85-15063

ISBN 0-917561-06-6   347.3063820269

First Edition

Printed in the United States of America

To Nan

Contents

Prologue

Seen through the eyes of Procter & Gamble, the United States of America is "the marketplace"—the arena of competition for the hearts and dollars of the American consumer. P&G has dominated the marketplace for decades; however, its success has not brought complacency but has fostered a zeal for ever-increasing sales and profits. Product lines developed within the company were the source of P&G's original growth, but expansion since World War II has come from buying companies with established products and, through P&G advertising and promotional genius, making those new products even more successful. Charmin paper towels, Duncan Hines food products and Folgers coffee are examples.

In the 1970s, P&G turned inward and developed a product of its own—a tampon that the company named Rely. Its revolutionary design and the use of superabsorbency materials made it an immediate success in the marketplace. Other tampon companies rushed superabsorbent tampons onto the market in a futile effort to stop the erosion of their sales. The outcome was an epidemic of an illness among menstruating women called Toxic Shock Syndrome (TSS). After close brushes with death, most TSS victims survive, but more than one hundred women have died since superabsorbent tampons became popular in 1977—and tampon-related TSS continues to claim its victims.

One of the women who died was Patricia Kehm, a twenty-five-year-old housewife and mother from Cedar Rapids, Iowa. This story focuses on her unnecessary death. But it is really about how a giant corporation responded when its most promising new product came under attack—the tactics that it employed when dealing, first, with the public health officials and, then, with the victims of TSS or their grieving families.

The lawsuit filed by the Kehm family permitted an inside look at Procter & Gamble in the form of hundreds of confidential P&G documents that recorded the thoughts and actions of company officials during the "Rely crisis"—documents that P&G fought to conceal from outsiders.

The tampon and Toxic Shock Syndrome controversy has produced its share of villains, both within and outside the government. But it has also produced some heroes—a team of young doctors at the Centers for Disease Control in Atlanta, Georgia, a young woman lawyer at the Food and Drug Administration and a relatively obscure microbiologist at New York University. They could neither be influenced nor intimidated by special interests. This book is dedicated in part to them.

The tampon companies can afford to spend millions of dollars just to promote their products on television alone. They are no less willing to spend whatever it takes in the defense of their products. Thus, this account is also dedicated to the few families who, like the Kehms, have had the courage to take the tampon companies all the way to a jury verdict—a few to win, others to be defeated by the vast resources of corporate giants like Procter & Gamble.

In telling the account of one TSS death victim, this book seeks to end the confusion about tampons and TSS, to expose a cover-up of important health information for menustruating women and to prod our government into effective action that can save the lives of those women who are otherwise doomed to die each year from Toxic Shock Syndrome.

PART
ONE

Innocent
Victims

1

"*You've really got to try Rely after the baby. They're so much better, you won't believe it.*"

Colleen Jones's advice to her sister, Pat Kehm.

Around 1:00 a.m. on September 5, 1980, Pat Kehm woke her husband, Mike, and told him she felt as if she were burning up. A short time later, she began vomiting at half-hour intervals. The vomiting continued into the morning. Pat was also running a fever and experiencing chills. Mike and Pat Kehm had two daughters: Andrea, who was two years old, and the baby, Katie. Neither parent wanted the little girls to catch what they assumed was the flu so Mike's mother came to pick up the baby, and Pat's sister, Colleen, took the older child.

The Kehms had just become Amway distributors and had planned a party for that evening. It was obvious to Mike that his wife was too ill to get anything ready so he stayed home from work. While Mike was doing the housekeeping and preparing for their guests, Pat started having severe diarrhea and was unable to keep anything down. Her fever fluctuated—at one point it was 101 degrees, at another 103 degrees.

Worried about her condition, Mike called their family doctor's office. The nurse said it sounded like the flu and to bring

3

Pat in the next morning if she didn't feel better. Around 5:00 or 5:30 that afternoon, Colleen brought Andrea back, but Mike's mother decided to keep the baby in view of Pat's deteriorating condition. Realizing that Pat could not recover in time for the Amway party, they decided to call it off.

Later that evening, Mike talked to his mother and told her that Pat was still vomiting and had diarrhea. His mother suggested that he should take Pat to the hospital. Mike agreed, and they arrived at the emergency room around 11:00 p.m.

There, Pat Kehm had her last chance to live. She was flushed and complained of a sore throat, and she vomited twice while at the hospital. Mike had never seen her this ill before. But the emergency room physician had not heard of TSS, and the treatment he prescribed was ineffective against the illness. He had misdiagnosed her condition as the flu and sent her home— something that occurred in hundreds of cases of TSS prior to the national publicity that was to accompany the withdrawal of Rely tampons from the market only two weeks later.

Pat Robinson was eighteen years old when she met Mike Kehm in 1973. Mike was a serious-looking young man who was already out of high school, had studied auto mechanics at a junior college and was employed as a service manager at a Pontiac dealership in Cedar Rapids, Iowa.

Two years out of high school and Mike was ready to settle down. Pat, on the other hand, was born settled down. Even though she was pretty and outgoing, she seemed much older and a little more old-fashioned than most high school seniors. She was not thinking about college or a long-term career but of children and a nice home. Pat assumed that when she married and became a mother, she would stay home with her children. This simplicity and selflessness were what Mike Kehm liked about Pat Robinson.

There were two reasons for Pat's aspirations. She was raised a Catholic in a conservative, industrial town in the Midwest and she had firsthand knowledge of what it was to have an unhappy marriage. Until her father's death, Pat's mother had endured a marriage to an alcoholic. Pat was certain that she wanted a reliable man, a man she could count on.

Mike Kehm was the all-American boy. He was clean-cut and polite to Pat's mother. He hardly drank at all. The Robinson family was elated when Pat and Mike Kehm became engaged. The only problem facing the couple was the fact that Mike was not a Catholic. Both families pretended that their children's different backgrounds were not important. Nonetheless, Mike's parents felt a twinge of sadness when they asked Mike: "Why is it that we're always expected to change?" He quietly and firmly told them he had decided to convert to Catholicism to "achieve complete harmony with Pat and our future children."

After their marriage in 1974, Pat worked as a secretary at St. Luke's Hospital and then at the city's Catholic hospital, Mercy. During this time, the Kehms bought a house. Pat quit her job just before the birth of her first child, Andrea, in 1978.

The loss of their second income created a financial crisis. Instead of going deeply into debt, the Kehms sold their house and moved in with Mrs. Robinson. A little over a year later, they were able to make a down payment on an older, less expensive home in a predominantly working-class neighborhood. It was in that two-story wood-frame house that the Kehms were the happiest.

Pat had an older brother, Ron, and two older sisters, Colleen Jones, nearest to Pat in age, and Jamie Lamon. Pat and Colleen were particularly close to one another and the two of them would usually spend Mondays together. Their mother would often join them.

Colleen had used Rely tampons since the winter of 1979–80. Her mother and mother-in-law had received free samples in the mail and had given them to Colleen. Colleen first told Pat about Rely tampons when her younger sister was pregnant with Katie.

She told Pat, "You've really got to try Rely after the baby.

They're so much better, you won't believe it." Pat's choice of tampons was Playtex, and she told her sister she really had no complaints with that brand.

Colleen continued to "kind of bug" Pat about using Rely. Pat resumed menstruating in July, approximately six weeks after the birth of Katie. Again, Colleen asked her sister if she had tried Rely yet, and Pat told her she had not.

Like many Catholics, Pat followed her own conscience and not the teachings of her church with regard to birth control. Six weeks after the birth of Katie, she saw her obstetrician-gynecologist, Gerald Shirk, M.D., to have an IUD reinserted. On August 27, 1980, Pat went back to Shirk for a pelvic examination and a checkup on the placement of the IUD. Shirk told her that the IUD was in good position, the pelvic examination was normal and she was in excellent health.

On August 29, 1980, Pat and her mother went shopping together. Remembering her sister urging her to try Rely, she picked up a box of Rely tampons and tossed it into her shopping cart. As she did so, Mrs. Robinson commented: "So you're going to try those dumb things." Pat's mother's reference was to tampons in general and not Rely. She had never used tampons, and her remark, growing out of her preference for sanitary napkins, was intended to put down all tampons in general. Mrs. Robinson, like her daughters, had not heard about Toxic Shock Syndrome.

As the summer of 1980 wore on, Pat Kehm was watching her baby, Katie, grow, and she was looking forward to the extra income she and her husband would make selling Amway products. In her diary entry of August 29, 1980, Pat wrote:

> "This past week was too busy for me. Had to go all over. Giant had a close-out sale. I spent $82.04 but got $164.08 worth of merch. We sell Amway. Hope we can build a $100,000 home in about 5 to 7 years. Katie sleeps from 10 to 7 now. Starting to take 4 hour naps. She smiles and laughs, especially while changing diapers. Both girls are so cute. I love our family."

Pat had told Becky Spore, her closest friend, about her and Mike's decision to become Amway dealers. As Becky later related, "Pat was so excited. They were doing okay with what Mike made at McGrath's, but Pat had this dream house in mind for the girls. She had drawn up the plans and estimated the costs. And now, with their distributorship, they were on their way." Becky's voice became quiet. "We talked about this two days before she died. You know, I'd never seen her happier."

On Labor Day, September 1, 1980, the Kehms took their daughters on a picnic. The next day, Pat's menstrual period would begin and she would follow her sister's advice and use Rely tampons for the first time.

On Wednesday, September 3, 1980, when Mike got home from work around 5:30 p.m., Pat had dinner ready for him. But after dinner, Pat asked her husband if he would take care of the girls; she felt "sluggish and kind of tired." She told him she ached a little bit and wanted to go to bed early, instead of waiting until 11:00, their usual bedtime. It was unusual for Pat not to feel well. When she worked at the two hospitals, she had never missed a single day due to health reasons.

The next day, Thursday, September 4, 1980, Mike Kehm got up at 6:00 a.m. Pat and the little girls always slept later. About 9:30 a.m., Mike received a call from his wife. "Pat asked if I'd come home to help her with the kids because she was feeling really bad. I told her to call me back if she wasn't feeling better in an hour because we were really busy. Pat called back in an hour to say that she was feeling good enough to get the kids lunch so I wasn't as worried."

Later that day, Colleen stopped by. Pat told her that she wasn't feeling well and on top of everything else she was having her period. Colleen asked her sister if she had tried Rely yet. "Pat said she was using one right now. And I asked her how she liked them. My question took her by surprise. Pat told me, 'I feel so bad that I haven't even noticed.' "

Mike got home from work around 5:30 and found that his wife had dinner ready for him, but Pat was so run-down that she went to bed early. That evening the vomiting and fever started, follwed by diarrhea the next day.

When Mike eventually took Pat to the hospital late Friday night, the emergency room doctor observed that Pat's throat was inflamed. Suspecting strep throat, he took a culture and sent it to the lab to see what would grow. He also gave her some antivomiting pills and a shot of penicillin—an antibiotic that is effective against many bacteria but not *Staphylococcus aureus*, or *Staph aureus* as it is often called—the bacteria present in all cases of TSS. Unaware of the cause of Pat Kehm's clinical symptoms, the emergency room physician sent her home with the suggestion that she see her doctor on Monday if she didn't "perk up."

On the way home from the emergency room the first circumstantial sign of shock appeared. Pat was dizzy when Mike took her back to the car, an indication that her brain cells were being deprived of the normal amount of oxygen. When they got home, Mike told his wife he was going to lie down on the couch in the living room so he could get some rest. He was so exhausted that he fell asleep before taking his clothes off. He was awakened at 8:30 a.m. on Saturday, September 6, 1980, by the sound of Pat talking to the family doctor's office on the telephone.

Pat was a fastidious person in her housekeeping and the care of her children as well as in her own personal hygiene. "Pat keeps Andrea so cleaned up and with every hair in place that she always looks like she could go to a studio and have her picture taken," her mother would often remark. So Mike was not surprised to find that Pat had risen earlier and somehow summoned the strength to take a bath so that she would look presentable at the doctor's office.

Dressing became another matter. Pat's legs were becoming discolored and sore. She couldn't bend her knees enough to put on her own blue jeans and needed Mike to help her get into a pair of his loose-fitting ones. Her condition was deteriorating so rapidly that she could not walk to the car; her husband had to carry her. Even though she wasn't exerting herself, she was panting, and Mike thought she must have a really bad case of flu. He would not hear of Toxic Shock Syndrome until later that day.

Pat's family doctor wasn't on call that Saturday, so she was scheduled to see his partner, John Jacobs, M.D., who was also a family practitioner. Jacobs was making his rounds at Mercy Hospital when Pat was carried by her husband into his nearby office. Pat wasn't strong enough to sit up at the doctor's office, and as she lay down on a couch, the nurse tried to take her blood pressure. By then, she had progressed so far into shock that the nurse could record no blood pressure by the conventional method of wrapping an inflatable cuff around the arm. Recognizing that a life and death struggle was going on in Pat's body, the nurse called Jacobs, who told her to call an ambulance to take Pat to Mercy Hospital. Both Kehms became frightened when the nurse told them an ambulance was coming to take Pat to the hospital—just two blocks away.

Dr. Richard Quetsch, a specialist in internal medicine, happened to be at Mercy Hospital to meet a patient in the emergency room when the ambulance brought Pat there. Quetsch, who did his residency training in internal medicine at the Mayo Clinic, is highly regarded by his peers in the Cedar Rapids medical community. As he walked through the corridor in the emergency area, Jacobs stopped him and asked him to help take care of Mrs. Kehm, whom he described as being seriously ill and in shock.

As he went to help, Quetsch thought to himself: There really aren't too many things that cause shock in women of that young age. He remembered a July 1980 *FDA Drug Bulletin* on Toxic Shock Syndrome, and he thought about a recent case he had treated that was probably a mild case of toxic shock, so he was considering TSS even before he reached Pat's side.

When he got there, he was struck by the appearance of her skin: "She was mottled, meaning different colors and in different parts of the body, a patchy discoloration of her trunk, particularly. Part of it was the kind of mottling that we often see with shock, with poor circulation getting to the skin, part pale, part purplish. But, in her case, there were some areas that were bright red—like first-degree sunburn would be, I guess."

Lois Sterenchuk, R.N., had the background and experience to be unflappable in her job. She had practiced her profession for more than thirty years. She had spent her entire nursing career at Mercy Hospital and served in all of the departments at one time or another before becoming house supervisor, a position she held at the time Pat was brought to the emergency room on September 6, 1980. Sterenchuk got a call from the charge nurse of the emergency room telling her that a patient had just come in who appeared to be very seriously ill and cyanotic. Sterenchuk asked if she should come and help out, and the charge nurse replied: "We are doing okay right now, but I just wanted to let you know that we have a patient who appears to be in serious condition."

About ten minutes later, the charge nurse called Sterenchuk again and said that the nurses in the emergency room had decided that she should come because the lady appeared to be "very critically ill."

When Sterenchuk arrived at the emergency room she understood the younger nurses' concern. Pat was having trouble breathing and was cyanotic. Her arms and legs were very dark, almost a bluish color. Sterenchuk's greatest worry was Pat's blood pressure: "The doctors were ordering many intravenous fluids, and trying to expand her fluid volume. She had a cut-down in her left ankle when I arrived. They wanted to get another IV started if we could, and I was able to get an IV started in her right arm."

Sterenchuk explained the procedure further: "A cut-down is when an excision is made in the skin and the vein is exposed and the vein is catheterized directly rather than by way of a needle through the skin—in Mrs. Kehm's case, a cut-down was necessary because her veins were pretty well collapsed and difficult to locate and to cannulate without direct exposure."

Sterenchuk described the scene as very hectic: "There were two trauma nurses there all the time I was there, two or three ambulance people were there, and they were assisting getting things that were being asked for, IV solutions, the nurses were monitoring her blood pressure, were fixing the medications, hanging IVs, providing oxygen, monitoring Pat's other vital signs, puncturing an artery to withdraw blood and sending it to the lab for tests and discussing why her pressure wouldn't come up."

At one point, Sterenchuk remembers something being said about "Toxic Shock Syndrome," then somebody saying: "We should probably get the tampon out." Sterenchuk removed a tampon from Pat and held it up to see if there was much blood on it. Since Pat was in such a pronounced state of shock, Sterenchuk was interested to know how heavily she was bleeding vaginally. She noticed there was very little, if any, blood on the tampon. Unaware of the possible significance of the tampon in Pat's illness and hearing no instructions from the doctors to do otherwise, Sterenchuk followed the hospital routine with such objects—she threw it in the waste receptacle in the emergency room.

Sterenchuk believes she had read an article on toxic shock prior to September 6, 1980, and her impression was that it seemed to be tied in with menstrual periods: "That was really all that I was familiar with."

In keeping with good hospital practice, Sterenchuk made an entry in the emergency room nursing notes showing that at 11:20 a.m. she had removed the tampon. The entry read: "Tampax removed by L. Sterenchuk, R.N."

At some point, the doctors found out that Pat had an IUD in place. Quetsch removed it and had it sent to the laboratory for bacterial analysis. *Staphylococcus aureus*, *E. Coli* and *Strep D* were eventually cultured from it.

Sterenchuk was with Pat continuously until 2:00 p.m., when she accompanied her patient to the intensive care unit and turned her care over to the ICU nurses. While Pat was still in the emergency room, she was having trouble breathing and was very apprehensive. Sterenchuk frequently told her: "Breath slowly and take it easy. We're doing everything we can to help you." The Kehm's parish priest, Father Donald Collins, was summoned. He did not see Pat nor give her last rites of the Catholic Church, however, for fear of the effect that it would have on her state of mind. At one point, Pat asked Sterenchuk: "Am I going to die?" The nurse told her: "Of course not." And she tried to reassure Pat that she was not in danger of dying.

There were times when the doctors entertained some hope that they might be able to save her. However, it became apparent that her blood pressure could not be maintained, and when she was transferred from the emergency room to intensive care, she was showing signs of pulmonary edema. In layman's terms, that means that there is more fluid being forced into the lungs by one side of the heart than the other side of the heart is able to pump out, and the lungs become like a sponge that is overloaded—the fluid just oozes out into the air spaces and the patient may drown in his own body fluids. The normal breathing rate of human beings is between 12 to 17 breaths per minute. Pat's respiratory rate was in the 40s. Normal heartbeat range is 60 to 80 heartbeats per minute. Pat's heartbeat was 160.

When her blood pressure was recorded by the special means of an electronic instrument called a Doppler, it was running in the 60s. The normal range for a person her age would be anywhere from 100 to 130 (systolic or upper reading) over 60 to 70 (diastolic or lower reading). To save her life, the doctors needed an upper reading of at least 90 and achieved it on two occasions only to have it fall back to the 80s after short periods. They could never even obtain a lower reading. Pat was put on a respirator when she was taken from the emergency room to intensive care. This only added to the problem of fluid accumulating in her lungs, so a mode called PEEP (standing for positive and expiratory pressure) was used in an attempt to keep the fluid pressure in the lungs from overcoming the air pressure in the air space so that the air space would be kept open. The risk of using PEEP is that if the air pressure is kept too high in an effort to keep fluid from the air space, the air pressure may exceed the pumping pressure of the heart, which stops the heart, and the patient dies.

The doctors and nurses worked for five and a half hours to save Pat's life, but she reached a point where she did drown in her own fluids, and her heart stopped. A Code Blue was signaled to alert the hospital personnel that a patient had stopped either heart or respiratory efforts. In Pat's case, a respirator was keeping her breathing going, but the monitor strip showed no heart reaction, and the doctors could not find a pulse or blood pressure. As Jacobs explains it, the lungs were not able to transfer oxygen to the arterial blood, and the heart was not receiving the necessary oxygen for its muscles to function, so the heart "just had no pumping capacity left." Repeated attempts were made to resuscitate Pat without success. Finally, five minutes after her heart had stopped beating, the doctors reluctantly pronounced her dead.

Mike Kehm had spent most of the time that day in the waiting room with his parents and Colleen. Every fifteen or twenty minutes or so, he had been permitted to see Pat. When she had first arrived at the hospital and was able to talk some, she complained to Mike, saying: "I can't breathe." Later, all she could do was just hold his hand while Mike offered encouragement. When Pat was moved into the intensive care unit, Jacobs and Quetsch came into the waiting room, and Mike asked them: "What's the worst thing I can expect?" Realizing that Pat had been on life support systems, he feared the possibility of brain or lung damage and mentioned that to the doctors. One of the doctors replied: "Well, those are all possibilities, but right now we are just trying to keep her alive." Mike was incredulous. It was the first time it hit him that she was that ill.

He spent the balance of the afternoon waiting and praying. At about a quarter to four in the afternoon, Mike was walking back to Pat's room when he ran into Pat's oldest sister, Jamie, in the hallway. He had not seen her earlier that day. Jamie was acting frantic at the nurses' station and she screamed at

Mike: "I think Pat's dead." Mike, disbelieving, told her: "Well, I'll go down and see, Jamie. Just relax." When he got to Pat's room, Jacobs told him that Pat had just died.

Pat's mother had not been called to the hospital and was under the impression that Pat had only a case of the flu. She could not believe what she was hearing when a weeping Colleen called her and said: "Mom, we've just lost our baby."

Mike numbly made arrangements for an autopsy and for the donation of Pat's corneas to the eye bank. Mike offered to let Pat's other organs be donated, but the doctors told him that, unlike the corneas, they had probably been damaged by the toxin and would be medically worthless.

He then went home to pick out some clothes for Pat's funeral. He noticed an opened box of Rely tampons on a shelf in the bathroom. Remembering the comments of the doctors at the hospital that his wife's illness might be associated with tampons, Mike picked up the box of Rely tampons and hurled it into the bathroom wastebasket. And he wept.

2

"Compared to traditional cotton and rayon tampons, everything about Rely is different—the shape, the material, the way it's made. Rely. It even absorbs the worry."

Message on box of Rely tampons.

On Tuesday, September 9, 1980, Mike Kehm buried his wife in a grave at Cedar Memorial Cemetery, one of those burial grounds like Forest Lawn that don't allow headstones—only simple plaques flush with the grass.

Eleven days after Pat Kehm's death, the federal government released a study that associated Rely tampons with an increased risk of Toxic Shock Syndrome. On Monday, September 22, 1980, Procter & Gamble announced that it was withdrawing its tampon product, Rely, from the marketplace. The next day, Tuesday, September 23, 1980, Dr. Jacobs met with Mike Kehm at his office near Mercy Hospital.

It is Jacobs's custom, when a patient in his care dies, to schedule a meeting with the family at his office. The purpose is to answer questions and to probe gently about their emotional well-being. Most importantly, he lets the family know he cares—one reason Jacobs has never been sued for mal-practice.

Jacobs asked Mike how he was getting along. The young widower told him that he was doing as well as he could under the circumstances. Jacobs then inquired if Mike had ever noticed a rash or redness on any part of Pat's body. Mike said that he had—that it was like a sunburn: when Mike had pressed on Pat's skin, it would turn white.

Jacobs told Mike that his wife had died of Toxic Shock Syndrome, a disease associated with Rely tampons. He explained that lab tests and the autopsy ruled out that Pat had died of anything else. He told Mike that they had done everything they could to save her. Mike agreed.

Mike didn't ask Jacobs about the failure of the Mercy Hospital emergency room physician to diagnose Pat's illness correctly the night before she died, and Jacobs didn't comment on that subject. The meeting ended with the doctor handing Mike a copy of Pat's death certificate and telling Mike to call him should he have any further questions at any time.

After the loss of his wife, Mike had made an appointment with his family lawyer to sign a will appointing his sister-in-law, Colleen Jones, as guardian for his little girls and leaving all of his property to them on his death. Mike told the lawyer what Jacobs had said about the cause of Pat's death, and they discussed the possibility of a products liability suit against P&G. No definite decision was made, partly because Mike got the impression that the family lawyer did not handle that type of litigation and would turn it over to someone else in his office.

The way Mike Kehm explained it to me when he came to my law office was that if he were going to have to deal with a lawyer who was a stranger to him, he figured he would pick one who he had heard was not afraid of taking on giant corporations. I was pleased at the compliment. My first impression of him was that the young man was deeply grieved by his wife's death and extremely bitter toward P&G. I detected a certain amount of vengeance. Yet, Mike seemed sincere when he spoke of taking P&G to court because he "owed it to Pat." I told him I would take the case and we discussed the question of fees. Mike chose a contingent fee instead of paying by the hour regardless of outcome. Under the contingent fee agreement, I would be paid one-third of whatever was collected from P&G, but Mike would have no legal fees if the suit were unsuccessful—just out of pocket expenses, something neither of us assumed would be very much.

At the time of our meeting, I had just opened my own firm, after having practiced with a relatively large firm for twenty-five years. This was the first big case to come into my office now that I was on my own. I was elated to get the case because I expected to do a good job for the Kehms, and frankly, I didn't think the publicity surrounding my handling of the case would hurt my new firm one bit.

After getting all the details of Pat's illness and death from Mike, I instructed him to look for any Rely tampons that might still be in his house and told him to refer anyone who asked him about the case to me.

After Mike left the office, I analyzed what needed to be done to get the case moving. It was obvious I had an excellent client in Mike Kehm—a clean-cut, nice-looking young man whose serious expression was enhanced by his eyeglasses. I wondered if he had been as serious and tense before his wife's death.

I needed to know where Pat Kehm had purchased the tampons. If they had been purchased at an Iowa-based store, suing the store, as well as P&G, would give us the option of trying the case in either state or federal court. If we sued only P&G in state court, federal law would allow P&G to have the case transferred to the federal court for trial. On balance, I preferred trying the case in state court for two reasons: state court allowed more opportunity to question prospective jurors to obtain their attitudes and prejudices, and a jury verdict did not have to be unanimous.

In the next few days, we interviewed friends and relatives of the Kehms and obtained a thorough factual background, but we were not able to establish where the Rely tampons had been purchased. Jean Robinson, Pat's mother, had been shopping with her when Pat bought the tampons, but she couldn't remember whether it had been Hy-Vee or Drug Town. Both were Iowa-based but there was no point alleging something that couldn't be proved, so the decision was made to prepare papers for filing in federal court.

My wife, Nan, and I have six children. Five of our children are girls, and although I felt I was normally attentive to the family, I could not recall paying any attention to the types of tampon brands that either my wife or our daughters used. I wondered if Mike had lacked the same interest until the day he returned to his home from the hospital and threw the Rely box in the wastebasket. I wanted to acquire a box of Rely tampons for possible use as a court exhibit but found that neither Nan nor our two youngest daughters still at home, Heather and Sara, had used the P&G product. By now, of course, Rely tampons were not available in stores. Stopping at a neighborhood pharmacy, I learned that the store had some in the back room that had not been returned to the supplier. I explained to the pharmacist that I wanted to buy one for evidentiary purposes only. The pharmacist gave me a box of Rely but would not let me pay for it, apparently in the belief that that would exonerate the pharmacy from any liability if the tampons caused injury or death. Although there was nothing illegal about the transaction, both the pharmacist and I acted like there was. Public interest in Rely tampons and TSS was then at its height. The pharmacist slipped the box of Rely into a plain brown sack and handed it to me.

At the office, I read the ironic slogan on the light blue box, "Rely, it even absorbs the worry." The choice of the brand name "Rely" reminded me of a law school course that dealt with fraud. One of the essential elements to make out a case for fraud was that the victim had to "rely" on the misrepresentation. The reasoning behind the law was that the victim had to trust what he was being told because, if he did not, the misrepresentation didn't influence his decision. P&G had picked for its tampon product a name that meant trust. That the customer could "rely" on the P&G tampon is what the brand name and all of the P&G promotional effort would be saying. Studying the innocent-looking box and its contents, I could not help but wonder what made Rely tampons sicken and kill some women: Was it a chemical or ingredient that acted as a poison? Was it some substance that was foreign to the tampon, like a contaminate? Or was it something basically faulty in the design that injured the vaginal area in some way?

At our next meeting, I told Mike Kehm that Mercy Hospital and the emergency room physician might be liable for negligence in failing to diagnose and treat Pat properly the night before she died. Mike said he was not interested in suing the hospital or the doctors no matter how the facts might develop. Remembering the flurry of activity that had attended the efforts of doctors and nurses at Mercy Hospital for five hours before Pat died, Mike explained that he could not bring himself to consider a suit for malpractice.

On September 29, 1980, I called Jacobs at his office and told him that I was representing Mike Kehm. I knew Jacobs from my past experience as a state legislator, and while we differed on political issues, I knew he was not afraid of controversy and hoped that would work to our advantage. With the deliberate intention of putting him at ease, I told Jacobs that Mike Kehm had no criticism of his efforts to save Pat's life and no intention of suing him or the other doctors, nurses or the hospital. I said that my client's case was strictly against Procter & Gamble as the manufacturer of Rely tampons. I told him that I was calling to verify that Pat had TSS, and Jacobs assured me that she did. I was surprised to learn that Jacobs did not know how Rely caused TSS—just that the Centers for Disease Control had found the connection with Rely a short time after Pat's death.

Aware that P&G had recalled its tampon product because of the government report, I had assumed that there would be a relatively simple explanation for the defect—like the botulism in the cans of soup that are recalled, or the steering defects that occur when insufficient pressure is used to tighten bolts at an automobile factory. Jacobs suggested that I contact Pat's gynecologist, Dr. Gerald Shirk, who was also my wife's doctor.

Since Jacobs had verified that Pat had died of TSS and her sister, Colleen Jones, told us Pat had been using Rely for her September menstrual period, I filed suit on September 30, 1980, against Procter & Gamble in federal district court in Cedar Rapids for $5 million in compensatory damages. I had suggested the sum of $3 million, but Mike, still grieving and bitter, ruled out that amount and requested the higher figure. So I filed the suit confident that Rely tampons were somehow responsible for Pat Kehm's death but knowing little more than that.

In early October 1980, I introduced myself to the Food and Drug Administration local agent as the lawyer for Pat Kehm's family. The agent already knew who Pat was. That same day he had been ordered by his superiors in Washington to investigate Pat Kehm's death, and he was glad that I had contacted him. It saved him the trouble of locating Mike Kehm for permission to interview his wife's doctors. I could authorize the doctors to release information to the agent.

The first question I asked the agent was: "What has the FDA found out was wrong with Rely?"

The agent said he didn't know. I was incredulous. I asked him why the FDA told P&G to recall Rely. He said all he knew was that there was a report issued a couple of weeks back in which Rely was singled out in TSS cases.

The Centers for Disease Control, known as the CDC, was established in Atlanta, Georgia, in 1946 to aid the states in the control of communicable diseases. Each week, it publishes its *Morbidity and Mortality Weekly Report*, called the *MMWR*, which, until recently, it distributed to some one hundred thousand doctors and others interested in public health who requested it.

The agent handed me a copy of an *MMWR*, a pamphlet about the size of a *Readers Digest* but only three or four pages

thick. The document was dated September 19, 1980. My
eyes fell on the words in the first paragraph:

> "In particular, there is an increased risk associated with
> the use of Rely tampons among TSS patients as com-
> pared with controls."

The agent told me he would like to talk to Jacobs for his
report. Back again at Jacobs's office, I asked the doctor if he
had learned anything more about why Rely caused TSS, and
Jacobs replied that he had not. He added that the first he had
heard of TSS was when Quetsch had mentioned it in the
emergency room the day Pat died.

After the agent obtained some data for the FDA questionnaire, we went to Shirk's office. Shirk told us that a bacterium
known as *Staphylococcus aureus* was believed to produce a toxin
that caused the illness. The bacteria, themselves, do not enter
the body, he pointed out, but rather, the toxin was produced
in the vagina and passed through the mucosal membrane and
into the body.

> "They think the tampons either dry out the vaginal wall
> or cause micro-ulcerations or lacerations to it or somehow
> disturb the mucosal membrane so as to permit the toxins
> to pass freely into the blood stream and poison the body,"
> Shirk explained.
>
> "You mean the tampon itself doesn't emit chemicals
> that poison the body or do something else to injure the
> woman?" I asked.
>
> "That's right. The staph bacteria have to be present or
> the woman won't get TSS. Tampons don't cause the
> problem by themselves. Otherwise, we'd have fifty mil-
> lion cases of TSS because that's how many women use
> tampons," the doctor pointed out.

Anticipating a claim by Proctor & Gamble that Pat Kehm
had been contributorily negligent, I asked:

> "Is it the woman's fault that she has that staph bacteria?
> In other words, is it a case of personal hygiene?"

"No," Shirk replied, "we all have bacteria in our orifices, such as the nose, mouth and, in the case of women, in the vagina. It's just a question of which bugs we happen to have, and there's no way of controlling that."

"What's the mucosal membrane, by the way?"

"In this case, we're talking about the vaginal wall," Shirk said. "Any lining of the skin that is always moist, such as the mouth or throat, stomach lining and so forth, is referred to as mucosal membrane."

"Are you fairly certain that injury to the mucosal membrane is the way Rely tampons cause TSS?"

"Frankly, no, it's just a theory. The puzzling thing is that tampons have been around for forty years or more and haven't caused TSS. The first reported cases were written up in 1978 and they involved children, some of whom were boys. I'd suggest you contact Rudy Galask in Iowa City. His specialty is microbiology of the vagina."

We thanked Shirk for seeing us on such short notice. Outside his office, I turned to the agent and said:

"I can understand the forty years angle since Rely is a new tampon. But what do you make of that business about boys getting TSS?"

The FDA agent merely shrugged his shoulders.

After returning to my office, I made an appointment for the next day to meet Dr. Rudolph Galask, who taught obstetrics and gynecology at the University of Iowa's College of Medicine.

The twenty-five mile trip from Cedar Rapids south to Iowa City, through yellowing cornfields ready for harvest and past the sprawling Coralville Lake Reservoir, was a pleasant one. At the University Hospitals and Clinics complex, I made my way through a labyrinth of corridors and irregular hallways, until I eventually located Galask's department. A secretary led me into a rather small office crammed with books, science magazines and papers.

"Jerry Shirk tells me that if anybody can tell me the tampon role in Toxic Shock Syndrome, you can, Doctor," I began.

Galask, a middle-aged man, smiled and said nothing to protest the accolade.

"Right now, we're in the theory stage. We know that the vagina can be an ideal culture medium for bacterial growth during menstruation because the menses provides nutrition in the form of blood and cellular debris, the pH level rises then and body temperature is next to optimal. If the menses flow is dammed up for long periods of time by superabsorbent tampons, which can be worn longer, then that could account for it, but frankly, I don't think anyone knows for sure what the answer is."

I asked:

"Could the tampons be contaminated with *Staphylococcus aureus* through mishandling by the manufacturer or distributor?"

"No, that isn't necessary since enough women have the *Staph aureus* as part of their normal vaginal flora to account for the several hundred cases of TSS that have been reported. Five to fifteen percent of women have *Staph aureus* present in the vagina at all times, and that means we're talking about five to fifteen million women and girls.

"By the way," Galask continued, " my 'star protégé,' Pat Schlievert, has been working on identifying the TSS toxin. I've been thinking of calling him to see how he is coming along."

"Any objection to calling him, now?" I asked.

Galask picked up the phone and dialed Schlievert at his laboratory at UCLA. He seemed excited by the information Pat Schlievert was relaying. When he hung up, he told me that Schlievert had just isolated the toxin that causes TSS, a pyrogenic exotoxin. I asked for an explanation.

"Pyrogenic means that it is fever producing and exotoxin means that it is excreted by the bacteria. There are two ways that bacteria can release toxin. One is by the bacteria manufacturing it within their cells and excreting it out like a waste by-product. Those are called exotoxins, and it's not known how many different exotoxins *Staph aureus* can produce.

"The other way toxins are released is when the cell dies and the toxin is in the wall of the cell and is released on the death of the cell. Those are called endotoxins," Galask explained.

I had assumed that there would be a simple cause and effect relationship regarding TSS and was just beginning to realize how complicated this matter was, but Galask assured me that it shouldn't be too long before we would have a scientific answer for the cause of TSS now that the toxin had been identified. Until then, however, we could not be certain as to the role of tampons in the development of the illness.

Knowing little more than I had before my meeting with Galask, I headed back to my office in Cedar Rapids, where I wanted to look over Mrs. Kehm's hospital records. About a third of the way through, I came across the typewritten report by Quetsch. Everything seemed to be in order until I reached the bottom of the page and read: "We were unable to establish whether she had a tampon in."

That was impossible. Mike had made it clear that his wife was having her menstrual period at the time of her illness and had been using Rely tampons. I knew P&G's attorney would pounce on that statement if Quetsch was adamant that there was no tampon removed from Pat Kehm in the emergency room. Reading further, I saw the notation that at 11:20 a.m. "Tampax removed by L. Sterenchuk, R.N." My God, I thought, this proves that a tampon was removed from Pat in the emergency room, but the nurse called it a Tampax and we're suing because of a Rely tampon.

I made arrangements to meet Lois Sterenchuk to find out why she had called the tampon a Tampax. Many people are less than enthusiastic about meeting with lawyers to discuss facts so I was pleased to find that Sterenchuk was more than happy to talk about Pat's case. Confident that everything had been done in the emergency room to save Pat Kehm's life, Sterenchuk did not need reassurances that the reason for the meeting was not to discuss possible malpractice by either the doctors or the nurses. Sterenchuk suggested that I meet her in the lounge of the main entrance of Mercy Hospital, after her duty shift ended.

I knew immediately that Sterenchuk's appearance would make her an excellent witness. Her face was that of a kind person, mature and motherly. While the stress of nursing causes many in her profession to become jaded, Sterenchuk was still obviously affected by the sudden and tragic death of Pat Kehm. She clearly wanted to help, yet I recognized that she was the type of person who would tell the truth, no matter what the consequences, and that the jury would recognize this characteristic about her. I hoped the truth would help my case.

I handed Sterenchuk a copy of the nurse's notes section of Pat Kehm's hospital records and pointed out the statement signed by her that a Tampax was removed from Mrs. Kehm. I was relieved when she said:

> "I call all tampons Tampax. That was the only tampon I used when I was menstruating. It's like calling all tissue Kleenex. I call all pads Kotex, too."
>
> "Do you know what kind of tampon you removed from Mrs. Kehm?"
>
> "No, I really don't. I've never seen one like that one. It was kind of like a bell-shaped tea bag with a string on the end of it."

I told the nurse that she had just described a Rely tampon. I explained that since Pat wasn't alive to tell the jury what kind of tampon she was using at the time she got sick, and that it might be a year or more before the case went to trial, I'd like to take her deposition soon to preserve her evidence. Sterenchuk agreed with me and we set a date for her deposition.

Well, that's one less hurdle to worry about, I thought as I left Mercy Hospital and headed for the office of Dr. Richard Quetsch, where there was more good news.

Quetsch said he had found in the nurse's notes section that the tampon had, in fact, been removed. "Apparently, one of the nurses had removed the tampon when I was out of the room or preoccupied," said the doctor.

"Well, that clears that problem up," I told him. "However, I noticed in the hospital records that the IUD which was removed from Mrs. Kehm had *Staph aureus* on it when it was cultured in the pathology department. Can they blame the IUD?"

"They may try, but you should be safe because if the IUD had been involved in the infection, then there should have been evidence in the uterus and the autopsy ruled out any infection at that point," Quetsch explained.

"The string hangs down into the vaginal vault while the coil of the IUD is in the uterus. The string could have picked up the staph in the vagina or the coil could have picked it up when it was removed, and this would explain why there was *Staph aureus* cultured from the IUD," he continued.

"I've heard that IUDs have been implicated in pelvic inflammatory disease." I was thinking of the Dalkon Shield litigation.

"Yes, that's true, but the kind of infections that you see with IUDs are very slow in developing," Quetsch pointed out. "Not three or four days like this young lady. I don't think this fits the picture of pelvic inflammatory disease. I don't know what tampons have to do with it other than what I've read. But I think Mrs. Kehm died of Toxic Shock Syndrome."

"Is that opinion based on reasonable medical certainty?" I asked, and then quickly added: "That doesn't mean absolute medical or scientific certainty under the law—just probability—you know, like if something has at least a 51 percent chance of happening, it's probable—that kind of probability."

"I think it's probable she had TSS, and while I don't know anything about the tampon's role in it, I've got to go with the government report that tampons have something to do with it," Quetsch concluded.

Later, in reviewing the September 19, 1980, *MMWR*, I noticed the name of Dr. Jeffrey Davis of the Department of Public Health of the state of Wisconsin. I reached Davis by telephone at his office in Madison. He was open and cooperative. In the course of our conversation, I learned that the September 19, 1980, *MMWR* was not the first report by the CDC on Toxic Shock Syndrome. Davis told me that there had been an issue published in May 1980 that described Toxic Shock Syndrome as a new entity that appeared to be associated with menstruation. Then, on June 27, 1980, the *MMWR* published the results of the first CDC study as well as the results of a Wisconsin Department of Public Health Study on TSS.

Both studies showed an association between tampon usage and TSS.

When I had been in Quetsch's office, the doctor had given me a copy of a document entitled *FDA Drug Bulletin*, July 1980, which contained a warning about tampons and TSS. I wondered if P & G had seen the FDA bulletin, because if their people had continued to sell Rely tampons without warning Pat Kehm and other women who got sick after July, it would make a stronger case for damages against P & G—maybe even permit a punitive damages award.

I asked Davis his opinion as to when P & G and the other tampon companies had learned of the June 27, 1980, *MMWR*. When Davis told me that P & G had found out before the *MMWR* was released, I asked him how he could be certain.

"Because I was there," Davis told me.

"All of the tampon manufacturers were invited to a meeting in Atlanta in the latter part of June, and the CDC people explained the results of the study to them, at that time."

"My client's wife died on September 6 of this year after starting to use Rely tampons for the first time on the 2nd of September. You mean to tell me that more than two months before that P&G knew of a government study that showed tampons had something to do with TSS?" I asked.

"There is no question about it. What's more, we told them about our study in Wisconsin, which reached the same conclusion. Since then, Utah and Oregon studies have also shown the same association."

What Davis said amazed me. I did not recall P&G or the other tampon companies making any public announcements or warnings about TSS until after Pat Kehm was already dead. Yet, I found it hard to believe that a reputable company like P&G, with all that could be lost in public image and credibility, could afford to be that callous. Why didn't they warn? I asked myself. What were they doing in the summer of 1980? Did they just stand by and let women die, and if they did, how could they still sleep at night? I resolved to find out.

3

"Tampons are really a very simple product."

P&G's response rejecting the FDA's request for ingredient
labeling, August 1, 1980.

The filing of a lawsuit is a declaration of war, I tell my clients—
whether they are doing the suing or being sued. And the first
rule of war is to know your enemy. At the onset, my knowledge of the Kehms's enemy was only that it sold Ivory—the
soap that floats and is 99&44/100 percent pure. From my
wife I learned that P&G made a host of items we used at
home—familiar items like Crest toothpaste and Tide laundry
detergent.

But I was especially interested in P&G's tampon product
and how it was developed. I found what I needed from four
disparate sources—research reports on P&G by stock analysts, FDA documents, the public library and P&G's own
files.

My investigation convinced me that P&G had manufactured an unsafe product, although I still didn't know how it
was defective. At the same time, it became clear that P&G
possessed incredible resources that could be used to disprove
that there was anything wrong with Rely.

The information that was gathered on P&G went into the Kehm trial notebook. I learned that Procter & Gamble, the manufacturer of the Rely tampons that Mike hurled into the wastebasket, was a relative latecomer to the tampon market. For nearly forty years, Tampax held a virtual monopoly on the sale of tampons while Kimberly-Clark dominated the sanitary napkin market. Increasing preference for tampons over napkins by young women, coupled with a growing youthful population, invited competition in the tampon market. The entry of Playtex and Kotex tampons in the market cut Tampax's share to 70 percent. It would drop to 42 percent by 1980 when Rely reached its peak. Sanitary napkin sales, however, were expanding at a rate slower than that of the population.

P&G had decided to develop a tampon product in the early sixties. It began, as it always does, with research—in this case by exploring women's attitudes about tampons. P&G found that women preferred tampons for their convenience and lack of visibility. The main dissatisfaction was that tampons bypassed, or leaked, more often than sanitary napkins.

Armed with that information, P&G technicians undertook to develop a tampon that would prevent bypass. The initial design consisted of cotton gauze sewn together in the compressed cylinder design similar to Tampax and the other brands. P&G then submitted its tampon to what it calls the win-buy test. In such tests, the P&G product, as well as competitors' brands, are placed in plain, unmarked packages and are given to selected consumers to be used on an alternate week by week basis. After a trial period, P&G interviews the consumers for their reactions to the P&G brand compared to competing brands. Women participating in the first P&G win-buy test on tampons preferred the P&G tampon. However, they did so primarily because the improved inserter that P&G had developed made it easier to use. It was not considered better in its actual functioning than those on the market.

P&G's development of a tampon product might have stalled at that point but for a significant change in television taboos in 1972. That year, the National Association of Broadcasters repealed its ban on television advertising of sanitary napkins, tampons and douche products. Overnight, the rules of marketing tampons were changed. Television, a medium that P&G dominates, would now allow a new tampon product to be quickly introduced to the consuming public—a major part of the formula P&G relied on to introduce and sell its other new products. To take advantage of TV marketing, work on a new P&G tampon began in earnest.

In designing its new tampon, P&G scientists rejected the traditional compressed cylindrical stick tampon design of other tampon brands and came up with a revolutionary construction. Its new tampon consisted of a tea-baglike sack filled with superabsorbent synthetic materials. Just as a tea bag lets water penetrate the sack, the tampon bag would allow the menses fluid to pass into the bag, where it would be soaked up and held by the absorbent materials inside. In addition to holding more fluid than the traditional cotton and rayon tampons, the synthetic materials in the P&G tampon bag would expand to fill the irregular space of the vaginal area and act as a dam. Bypass would be prevented—something the other tampons with their regular shape could not do. Women could leave them in place for longer periods without the fear of embarrassment. Rely truly "absorbed the worry."

While its engineers were designing the new tampon, P&G marketing people were spending equal effort selecting a name for it. P&G knew that the right product name would be vital to the success of their mass-marketed product. What P&G looks for in a product name was set out by P&G group vice president Charles Fullgraf during testimony in an unsuccessful lawsuit P&G had filed against Johnson & Johnson in 1979. P&G contended that the name of Johnson & Johnson's new tampon, "Assure," was deceptively similar to the name of P&G's deodorant "Sure." Fullgraf testified:

"We are looking for names that are as simple as possible, as memorable as possible. If we can find names that have a positive connotation for the given product area, we are interested in that. Failing in that, we are interested in finding names that are neutral and which we can make mean what we want them to mean over a period of time with sustained advertising."

"Sure" was Fullgraf's choice for the name of P&G's new tampon. Fortunately for P&G, Fullgraf's point of view did not prevail. Had it, P&G's "Sure" brand of deodorant would have been irreparably damaged by the controversy that would later surround Rely tampons. Fear of such a domino effect was the very reason P&G selected a new brand name for its tampon.

Martin Cannon, P&G's official in charge of developing Rely, said the selection of the name Rely was a result of testing that demonstrated it to be a name that was easy to recall and understand. Rely means "to depend," "to trust," and "to lean on with confidence, as when satisfied of the truth." Those dictionary definitions fit the positive connotation that P&G desired in a product name. Women could rely on the tampon sold by P&G—they could trust it. And, to the trustworthy sounding name of Rely for its tampon, P&G added a slogan that built on that theme of trust and security: "It even absorbs the worry."

Television would be a key to P&G's introduction of Rely to the marketplace. In 1980, nobody spent money on commercial television like Procter & Gamble. Of the $649 million P&G allocated for advertising in 1980, the year of Pat Kehm's death, $496 million, nearly half a billion dollars, was spent for commercial sponsorship of television shows. About $250 million are spent for the thirteen soap operas P&G sponsors. Unlike its less fortunate competitors, P&G produces six of the "soaps" and is able to spend advertising dollars on its own shows. The public doesn't appreciate the magnitude of P&G T.V. advertising because the commercials usually mention only the product's name, like Crest, for example, without mentioning P&G.

It is ironic that while P&G is responsible for what may be considered some of the more licentious T.V. programs, it has been praised from the pulpit by Jerry Falwell, leader of the Moral Majority. As spokesman for the Coalition for Better Television, Falwell announced in 1981 that television shows would be monitored for sex and profanity content, and he threatened boycotts against the producers or sponsors of television shows that violated the standards set by his coalition. P&G earned Falwell's gratitude, however, when its then company chairman, Owen Butler, in a June 1981 speech to the Academy of Television Arts and Sciences, pledged P&G's support for efforts to clean up television.

Falwell was aglow with kind words for Procter & Gamble: "Until P&G's speech, we didn't know so many advertisers agreed with us . . . it is unfortunate the networks are so out of touch with the public." Critics of P&G's moral support for the Moral Majority accused the giant soap company of "selling the advertising industry down the river." Knowledgeable observers claimed P&G's boycott fears were not due to the attacks on its sponsorship of prime-time programing but, instead, arose from anxiety that the focus of the criticism would shift to the daytime soaps in which P&G had a much greater financial stake. Falwell's gratitude over P&G's endorsement of his pressure group's goals, however, was such that he granted the giant soap company a reprieve:

> "P&G has taken such a massive step that we have to give them some time to clean up daytime."

P&G did not depend solely on its television muscle, however, to promote the sale of Rely. It employed its "force-trial" method, which introduces customers to a new P&G product by providing free samples, reduced price coupons or discount prices. In Rely's case, P&G sent out millions of free samples through the mail.

After P&G had developed its revolutionary tea-bag tampon, it began test marketing—first in Fort Wayne, Indiana, in 1974, and the following year in Rochester, New York. If a P&G product meets with consumer acceptance in test mar-

keting, then a "roll-out" occurs with the product being introduced in regional stages rather than throughout the entire
country at once. With Rely tampons, the roll-out began on the
West Coast, moved to the Southwest, then through the Middle West, down to the Southeast and, finally, finished in the
Northeast part of the United States. By rolling out a product
in successive stages, P&G is able to concentrate a saturation
promotion campaign in the region in which the product is being
introduced. If problems develop, the regional campaigning can
be changed or abandoned without incurring the expense of a
national campaign.

P&G would contend that exhaustive safety testing was done
on Rely before it was sold to women in Fort Wayne—in line
with its claim that each P&G product must be found safe
before it is first sold. But there was no microbiological testing
of Rely before selling began in Fort Wayne and only limited
microbiological testing later. Although Fullgraf had admitted
in the Johnson & Johnson lawsuit that the vagina was subject
to a higher level of infection and bacterial invasion than any
orther organ of the body, P&G, prior to marketing Rely, didn't
perform simple laboratory tests to see what bacteria found in
the vagina would do to the components of its tampon and what
effect such components would have on the bacteria
P&G set up a so-called Scientific Advisory Group for Rely
but it did not have a microbiologist on it.

Testing had been done to determine what effect Rely components might have in causing allergy reactions or skin irritations. But it was in P&G's interest, before spending millions
of dollars to promote Rely, to make certain that the product
wouldn't be rejected by the consumer because of dermatolog-
ical effects that it caused.

The Rely components were fed to rats and no adverse effects were noted. But in one test, the components placed inside
the vaginas of rats caused the vaginal tissues to become irritated with redness, swelling and lesions. P&G attributed this
to the method of the test and not the effect of the components.
Testing on animals for skin irritations outside the vagina pro-

duced no adverse results, so P&G proceeded in 1973 to employ Dr. Tommy Evans, then chairman of the department of obstetrics and gynecology at Wayne State University, to set up a clinical evaluation of women who would use Rely tampons.

Evans was a longtime consultant of P&G, having been on an annual retainer since 1963. He projects the image of a nice guy somewhat embarrassed by his many honors and titles in the field of obstetrics and gynecology, one of which was serving as editor of *Ob-Gyn News*. But Evans also has the distinction of having approved two products that were ultimately withdrawn from the marketplace under a cloud of suspicion—Rely tampons and the drug Bendectin. The latter, a pill for morning sickness during pregnancy, was withdrawn after being linked to birth defects, although subsequently, different juries have reached contradictory verdicts on its responsibility for the birth defects.

Evans, as part of a four-man team, was in charge of a clinical study of 118 women, half of whom used Rely tampons while the other half used Tampax. Evans's team pronounced Rely safe for marketing because it showed no material difference from Tampax in the type of bacteria found in the vagina during tampon use. On the basis of this limited clinical evaluation of only 43 women using a new product (32 dropped out of the study), millions of tampons were distributed and sold to American women.

Curiously, in the report to P&G on their clinical testing of Rely, Evans, and two of the other three medical doctors, advised against contacting the FDA about the new product. Dr. Richard Stoughton, of Duluth, Minnesota, apparently did not subscribe to this approach, and he, alone, refused to sign that portion of the report approving Rely for test marketing without first contacting the FDA.

P&G continued intermittent testing of Rely up to the time of the TSS controversy in 1980. But the testing ignored warnings from P&G's own researchers or consultants. In 1976, Gordon Flynn, a P&G consultant and professor of pharmaceutics at the University of Michigan, told P&G he worried about the fact that the tampon had the ability to make the vaginal surface alkaline, "which would lead to bacterial colonization and infection." He suggested P&G seek ways to preserve the acidic character of the environment. P&G ignored his recommendation.

In 1972, Joyce Davis, a scientist from Hill Top Research Laboratories, recommended an expanded bacteriological study of Rely if the study that she was working on showed an average pH difference of at least one unit between the examination during menstruation, and an exam either before or after the menstrual period. Her study turned up such a pH difference, yet the recommended bacteriological studies were not carried out. In 1974, a Rely safety summary analyzing long-term effects of tampon use said that data to support the absence of chronic or long-term effects would probably be judged inadequate in an adversary proceeding.

On February, 28, 1975, P&G scientist R. B. Drotman outlined "a list of possible areas of attack on the safety of Rely." These included: "Rely has an effect on the bacterial flora of the vagina"; "Menses is rich in enzyme and this changes the chemical nature of leachable materials [from Rely]"; "The materials will be absorbed by the vagina and enter the systemic circulation with different materials leached at different vaginal pHs"; "There are substances that are part of Rely that result in undue vaginal irritation and/or sensitization."

Years later, Drotman claimed, in a TSS lawsuit P&G defended in Missouri, that the items on the list did not represent actual dangers in his opinion but that he was merely being a devil's advocate and listing all theoretical areas that some outsider might raise as a criticism. Nonetheless, at the time he wrote his memo, P&G had already sold the product to women in test markets and proceeded to launch its national roll-out of Rely without conducting scientific tests to determine the validity of Drotman's "attacks on the safety of Rely."

P&G's test marketing of Rely in Fort Wayne, Indiana, in 1974 was uneventful and successful. The test marketing that began in Rochester, New York, in February 1975 was a different story. In July of that year, the *Rochester Patriot* reported that Rochester women were being used as guinea pigs by P&G for a new tampon called Rely that contained polyurethane. The *Patriot* claimed polyurethane had been shown to cause cancer in laboratory animals.

A group of Rochester women, lead by a consumer activist, Judy Brayman-Lipson, were outraged at being guinea pigs for a relatively untested product. When Brayman-Lipson, president of the Empire State Consumers Association, wrote to P&G about the polyurethane issue, P&G cited four years of safety testing on Rely components. P&G refused to release this data, however.

P&G did agree to commission a review of the test data by Dr. Henry Thiede, chairman of the department of obstetrics and gynecology at the University of Rochester. The company's reply to Brayman-Lipson concluded with a promise that Dr. Thiede ". . . has agreed to review our safety and performance data on Rely and then we'll be prepared to answer any medical questions you or your associates may have concerning this product."

That was on August 15, 1975. Although Brayman-Lipson had a friendly relationship with Thiede (her husband was a medical colleague in Rochester with a specialty in internal medicine), Thiede did not contact Brayman-Lipson as P&G had promised, and he repeatedly refused to talk about his report to P&G with either the *Patriot* or Brayman-Lipson. The Thiede report has never been made public. P&G claims it never received a report.

In response to an inquiry by the *National Publication Media and Consumer*, P&G contended that the *Patriot* articles about the polyurethane controversy were inaccurate and harmfully misleading. According to P&G, the tests on polyurethane had shown that tumors are induced only when the polyurethane is surgically implanted within the body of laboratory animals. The *Patriot* fired back: "But the company neglected to mention that the tests, conducted by such well-known research centers as the National Cancer Institute and the University of Tennessee, have also found the tumor-causing properties to be related to chemical decomposition of polyurethane in addition to its surgical implantation."

During the Rochester controversy surrounding the use of polyurethane, P&G refused to divulge the ingredients of Rely because "trade secrets would be involved."

On November 19, 1975, the *Patriot* reported that an FDA compliance officer, Kurt Hirchma, advised that the Rely tampon would come under investigation by the FDA and that "it now appears that Procter & Gamble had not tested Rely sufficiently before releasing it to the Rochester market." Hirchma also indicated that the labeling on the Rely package was not in compliance with federal regulations. The newspaper claimed that the Monroe County Health Department had indicated its interest in investigating consumer complaints about Rely and that Delta Laboratories, an independent public interest laboratory, had said that it had begun tests of Rely.

At that point, P&G threw in the towel in Rochester and announced that it had decided to redesign the tampon and replace the polyurethane in Rely with a cellulose product. While still maintaining that polyurethane was safe, P&G said the reason for the change was that the company feared continued use of polyurethane would negatively affect sales. Interestingly, P&G continued to ship Rely tampons with polyurethane to Fort Wayne until the supply was used up. A P&G memo indicates that this was done because there had been no controversy in that area.

Wittingly or not, the women of Rochester and Fort Wayne served as laboratory animals in Procter & Gamble's marketing experiment of its new and revolutionary tampon. Of course, the experiments Procter & Gamble conducted in Rochester and Fort Wayne were primarily designed to determine consumer acceptance of Rely as a substitute for the brand women had been using—not to see if health problems were created by Rely. But the extended test marketing in those cities did have the side benefit of registering the volume of health complaints.

When controversy persisted over the use of polyurethane as a possible carcinogen, P&G eventually replaced it—but not before thousands of Rochester and Fort Wayne women were exposed to its effects. And when the women in the test markets complained of difficulty in dislodging the tampon because the string would often break, P&G replaced it with a stronger string. The women in the test markets were human guinea pigs for a product that required no prior governmental approval before being sold and distributed to other guinea pigs— the rest of the female population who preferred tampons over napkins during menstruation. And, like real guinea pigs, they did not know that they were taking part in an experiment.

Procter & Gamble was willing to spend millions of dollars to advertise and promote. But when it came to compensating the few women who knowingly participated in Rely testing, P&G was more careful with its dollars. In 1976, P&G contacted Dr. D. P. Schwartz of the Albany Medical College at Union University to obtain women volunteers for a study. The women would wear Rely tampons made with a different synthetic foam to replace the polyurethane that had raised objections from Rochester women. Schwartz had proposed paying each volunteer $500 for her participation in an eight-month study, but P&G protested that the sum was too high. A company that would spend $600 million in annual television advertising in 1980, plus $11 million just to mail out free samples of Rely, balked at paying women $14.53 per week to women who would test a new product that would be placed inside their bodies.

By 1980, P&G was spending at a rate of $15 million annually in advertising Rely, which was more than the combined spending of the other tampon companies. The roll-out was an astounding success from P&G's standpoint. Starting at a virtual zero share of the market in 1978, P&G's Rely jumped to 12 percent of the national market share in the first quarter of 1980 and to a 20 percent share in the second quarter of 1980. In the regions where Rely had been introduced early in the roll-out, the market share had climbed higher than 25 percent.

The Rely gains came at the expense of the other four tampon companies. Tampax, still the leader, dropped as low as 42 percent in the summer of 1980. A few years earlier, it had been 90 percent. Shortly after Rely was withdrawn, the consensus of research analysts at one large stock brokerage firm was that: "Clearly, Rely had an excellent chance of replacing Tampax as the leading tampon by 1981 or 1982."

As 1979 came to a close, the team of P&G personnel responsible for the development and marketing of Rely could take satisfaction in their accomplishments. They had created a product that increasing numbers of women were buying. The continued roll-out, together with the advertising and force-trial methods, was certain to keep Rely's "momentum in the marketplace."

And the heavy advertising and promotion campaign of Rely would be maintained as the competition between the super-absorbent tampons continued to intensify.

One of the free sample boxes of Rely would be mailed to Pat Kehm's mother, Mrs. Jean Robinson. She would give it to Pat's sister, Colleen, who liked it so much, that she became a regular user—until Pat's death in September of 1980. Now she buys no product with a P&G label on it.

4

"Next it will be Pampers"

The reaction of a P&G official upon learning that Rely
was linked to TSS.

The picture of Dr. James Kennedy Todd in *People* magazine
reminded me of the handsome young doctors portrayed in
P&G soaps. But Todd, of the Children's Hospital of Denver,
was the real thing. In person I found Todd to be slightly con-
descending. At the same time, he was a highly competent pe-
diatrician specializing in infectious diseases.

Todd earned his bachelor's degree in microbiology and a
medical doctorate at the University of Michigan. Another six
years were spent in internships and residency at Ann Arbor
before his additional residency at the nationally recognized
Children's Hospital of Denver. Todd joined the staff in 1973
and worked up to head of its infectious disease department.
He also held a teaching position with the medical school of the
University of Colorado.

In 1975, a critically ill sixteen-year-old boy had come under
Todd's care. His symptoms included fever, vomiting, diarrhea, a sunburn-like rash on his body, and he was in deep
shock. Within a few days of the boy's hospitalization, Todd
noticed marked peeling of the skin on his palms and soles.
Bacteria in the blood might have explained the illness, but lab

tests showed none present. The youngster's only source of illness was a small abscess on his buttock. The case puzzled Todd. No disease he had heard of matched the boy's set of symptoms. Todd didn't know what the illness was, but he knew it was different from anything he had previously encountered or read about.

During the next two years, Todd saw a total of seven children with the same symptoms. Their ages ranged from eight to seventeen years of age. One died, one had gangrene of the toes and the others recovered. The bacterium, *Staphylococcus aureus*, was found in either the patient's nose, throat, vagina or in an abscess in the body, but it was not found in the blood. Todd surmised that the bacteria produced a toxin that entered the bloodstream and caused the illness. Todd coined the name "Toxic Shock Syndrome" for the newly described illness. Scientists use "syndrome" for an illness that has a consistent collection of clinical symptoms but no proven cause.

In 1978, the *Lancet*, a British scientific journal, published an article by Todd describing the illness. Though this article established Toxic Shock Syndrome as the name for the illness and Todd as the authority on it, it received little attention in the United States until the winter of 1979–80, when public health departments began receiving reports of young women becoming seriously ill and, in some cases, dying from Toxic Shock Syndrome.

Todd later admitted he had missed the possibility of a connection between Toxic Shock Syndrome and tampon usage. Four of Todd's original seven child cases were menstruating females, two of whom had vaginitis. Todd eventually learned that at least three of the girls used tampons.

Public health officials began to suspect a menstruation connection with TSS in early 1980. Among them were Dr. Jeffrey P. Davis, state epidemiologist for Wisconsin, and Dr. P. Joan Chesney, chief of the Infectious Disease Division of the University of Wisconsin School of Medicine. In the short span of four days in December 1979, Chesney learned of three cases of TSS while Todd had seen only seven cases over a two-year period. Recognizing a possible outbreak in the making, Davis interviewed the three victims and found some interesting similarities. For one thing, each had fallen ill during menstruation. For another, their same illness had occurred during previous menstrual periods.

Reports of other cases in Wisconsin started to come in with alacrity, and Davis soon had 35 cases under investigation. Of that number, 34 (or 97 percent) had been using tampons when they became ill. The sole, nontampon-using victim had an abscess on her heel.

On January 31, 1980, Davis wrote to 3,500 doctors in Wisconsin to alert them to the clinical symptoms of Toxic Shock Syndrome and to warn of its possible association with menses and staph infection. At about the same time, Andrew Dean, epidemiologist for the state of Minnesota, notified the Centers for Disease Control of the spread of the newly recognized syndrome in his state. Davis of Wisconsin followed suit, as did the state epidemiologist for Illinois. As a result of the Davis letter to doctors in Wisconsin, the *Milwaukee Journal* heard about this recently identified health problem and, on February 14, 1980, published the first news story on TSS, but the story made no mention of tampons.

A vital unit of the CDC is the Epidemic Intelligence Service, known as EIS. Established in 1951 as a mobile unit, it investigates outbreaks of disease when the problem is too big for local or state public health departments. It functions somewhat in the manner of a branch of the military service with the ordinary tour of duty lasting two years. The physicians are not actually members of the military, but they serve in positions that have a recognized equivalent rank, with corresponding pay, to military officers. Duty with the EIS is considered excellent training in public health and epidemiology for the young doctors.

Two of the young EIS officers in 1980 who were prominent in the TSS investigation were Dr. Kathryn Shands and Dr. Bruce Dan. Shands obtained her bachelor of science degree at Cornell University, her medical degree from Boston Univer-

sity and served her internship and residency in pediatrics at
Massachusetts General Hospital. Her colleague, Dan, received his bachelor of science at M.I.T. and pursued graduate
studies at Purdue and M.I.T. in biomedical engineering, the
engineering aspects of the biology of medicine. He then earned
his M.D. from Vanderbilt Medical School, where he also served
his internship and residency in internal medicine. Dan followed his residency work with postdoctoral studies in infectious disease. Dan was board certified in internal medicine.

When reports reached the CDC of the potential epidemic
in toxic shock cases, Shands was assigned to investigate the
problem. In February of 1980, she contacted James Todd in
Denver to tell him of these reports and ask his advice. She told
Todd that the illness seemed to occur primarily in young
women, and there was a suspicion among three state epidemiologists in the Middle West that there might be a menstrual
association. With Todd's help, Shands and the other doctors
at the CDC established a strict case definition of Toxic Shock
Syndrome to be used for epidemiological purposes—to determine the extent of the epidemic and its spread-rate.

The case definition of TSS required that the patient have
certain clinical findings: a fever of 102 degrees Fahrenheit or
higher, a sunburnlike rash on the skin, hypotension (low blood
pressure) and, within one to two weeks after the onset of the
illness, desquamation—a sloughing off or peeling of the skin,
particularly on the hands and feet. In addition, the case definition required there be involvement of at least three body
systems. One of these systems would usually be the gastroin-
testinal tract, and the patient would experience vomiting and
excessive diarrhea.

The CDC had another purpose in formulating a strict case
definition. It intended to conduct a statistical study of TSS
victims in the hope of finding what medical doctors call the
etiology, or cause, of the illness. In order to be able to draw
valid conclusions from the statistical study, it was imperative
that only bona fide TSS cases be included in the study. Even
a probable TSS case would be excluded if one or more clinical
symptoms of the strict definition were not present. This would

avoid what is known as diagnostic bias—a mistake in diagnosis. The statistical type of study of TSS that the CDC decided to conduct in early June 1980 is known as a retrospective case control study. A CDC task force, with Shands as director and Dan as deputy director, collected reports on cases of TSS victims. They limited their study to menstruating women because the overwhelming majority of TSS victims were menstruating when they became ill. They suspected that menstruation or menstrual products played some key role. The cases of TSS that did not occur in menstruating women had an obvious site of infection, such as an abscess, to explain the source of the illness. The cases of menstruating women did not.

After identifying fifty-two verified cases of TSS in menstruating women, the task force set up a matching control group, consisting of a women friend of each case, who was within three years of her age. Both the cases and the controls were asked to answer a detailed questionnaire in an attempt to see what differences there might be between the two groups that could explain why the cases got TSS.

The CDC task force had considered and then rejected doing a prospective study, which would have involved a large group of persons, identifying their traits and habits and waiting for TSS to occur. The prospective study would have been the CDC's choice of methodology because it would have had the advantage of avoiding possible diagnostic and memory error inherent in recalling past events. But it could have taken a year or more to complete, and in June of 1980, women were dying of TSS and the CDC doctors did not want to wait a year or more to find out why. In addition, the CDC doctors realized that since the incidence of TSS was low—estimates ran from 3 to 15 cases per 100,000 people—it would involve enrolling an unmanageable group of more than a million menstruating women to be sure of turning up the minimum 50 TSS cases they wanted to study.

On May 23, 1980, the CDC had published its first *MMWR* on TSS. It had described the symptoms and noted that of the 55 cases reported since the preceding October 1, 7 deaths had occurred for a fatality ratio of 13 percent. TSS cases and deaths were being reported with increasing frequency. So the CDC decided it had to act fast—even if it meant absolute scientific certainty was sacrificed.

The questionnaire used by the CDC in its study asked both cases and controls a number of personal questions about their sexual activities, menstruation and their use of tampons and sanitary napkins during an "index period." In the case group, the "index period" was the menstrual period when they contracted TSS. Women in the control group were asked questions about their most recent period in order to avoid the possibility of memory error on the control's part.

Although the women in the case group were searching further back in time, the EIS officers reasoned that the illness had such an impact on the victims that their memory of things during the illness would be indelibly etched in their minds. As Bruce Dan noted:

> "Everybody my age remembers what they were doing when they heard the news of John F. Kennedy's assassination—our parents remember what they were doing when Pearl Harbor was attacked."

While the task force was conducting its study, Shands contacted all tampon manufacturers. On June 13, 1980, she reached P&G's associate director with responsibility for product safety, Gordon Hassing, by telephone and briefed him generally on TSS and the CDC study. She told him she was contacting tampon manufacturers to find out what they knew about the prevalence of tampon usage, explaining that TSS seemed associated in some way with menstruation and the CDC was looking at all menstrual factors. Hassing asked her if there was any evidence of a tampon connection. She replied that it was too early to tell. Shands confided to Hassing that she had told a *Los Angeles Times* reporter there were no data yet suggesting the possibility of a link with TSS only to find out a few days later that the reporter had discovered ten cases of TSS in Los Angeles, all involving women using tampons.

Following his telephone conversation with Shands, Hassing received a call from Keith Colborn, manager of a P&G factory located in Iowa City, Iowa. Colborn told Hassing that a professor at University of Iowa Hospitals was studying Rely tampons for chemical impurities. Colborn had learned of it from a P&G employee whose husband worked as a laboratory technician for the professor. Hassing told Colborn to have the husband convey the message that "P&G would be very interested in the results of his work and would like to help the professor." Colborn then told Hassing that the professor was linking tampons to several recent severe illnesses requiring hospitalization and "of other cases around the country where even a death had occurred."

After speaking to Colborn, Hassing dictated a memo about the call to a P&G colleague. He concluded:

> "This suggests to me that they may be dealing with several cases of toxic shock syndrome.
>
> "Currently, I propose to wait to see if the professor calls me. There are several other options for being more aggressive in getting information about who the professor is and what the specific work is, but I view these options now as raising too high a profile."

On June 19, 1980, an anxious Hassing and his boss, Owen Carter, called Shands to find out the status of the CDC study. Shands told them the study was "almost complete," with only three or four cases left to process, and that it had taken nine doctors over four days to make the investigation. When they pressed her for the results of the study, Shands gave them the bad news:

> "In cases we have analyzed, one hundred percent of the women had used tampons exclusively!"

Shands then told the stunned P&G officials that the CDC would like to hold a briefing with tampon manufacturers and FDA representatives the following week when the study was finished.

When the final computer printouts of the study were delivered to Shands and the other task-force doctors, their suspicions were confirmed. Although about 30 percent of women in America used napkins during their menstrual periods, not one of the TSS victims in the study had. Instead, every one of the victims of TSS had used tampons at the time she became ill. Among the controls, however, 43 of the 50 (86 percent) used tampons. In the science of statistics, such a difference in tampon usage between case and control is deemed statistically significant—meaning that it is improbable that the association of tampons with TSS victims was a coincidence or a result of chance.

At about the same time the CDC study was completed, reports of separate studies from Wisconsin and Utah both showed the same results. In the Wisconsin study, 34 of 35 TSS patients (97 percent) used tampons during every menstrual period compared to 71 of 93 controls (76 percent)—a statistically significant difference. The Utah study was too small to be statistically significant, but all twelve of the TSS patients (100 percent) used tampons. Eventually, the Utah study would be expanded to 29 TSS cases and 91 controls, which made the results statistically significant. All 29 TSS cases were tampon users (100 percent) compared to 70 of 91 controls (77 percent). All three studies used a different method of selecting for the controls. The CDC study used friends, the Utah study used neighbors and the Wisconsin study used persons who visited the same gynecologic clinic.

On June 20, 1980, Shands called Hassing and proposed that the briefing be held in Atlanta on Wednesday, June 25, 1980, with the CDC, FDA and all tampon manufacturers present. It would be preceded on Tuesday by private meetings with each tampon company.

Following that telephone conference, a sober Hassing wrote to other P&G officials:

"At this point, it is beginning to look like there is a possibility that tampons could be involved in the development of TSS. It will also be very difficult to show that they are not involved without more data. . . . . There is the possibility of an eventual highly adverse publicity situation concerning the tampon category at some point in the future."

On June 24, 1980, the CDC task force and FDA representatives met privately with each of the tampon companies. P&G answered the CDC doctors' questions about the marketing history of Rely, its construction and key ingredients. At the briefing for all manufacturers the next day, the CDC furnished data from all three studies, as well as the questionnaires and computer tapes used in the CDC study.

On his return from Atlanta, Hassing wrote other P&G officials that the CDC data collected by the three studies were consistent and that the biostatistical approach used in the three studies was correct. Mindful of the possibility of adverse publicity and in anticipation of the soon-to-be released *MMWR* containing the three studies, Hassing noted: ". . . we will work today on public relations statements." What he had in mind was set out in a memo he dictated the day before he left for the Atlanta meeting on June 24, 1980:

> "We will hope to position Rely as *'part of the pack*,' i.e., keep this problem [TSS] only theoretically associated with the category [Rely]."

An equally apprehensive appraisal of the situation appears in a memo of P&G vice president James M. Edwards:

> "We are persuaded by the CDC and other data that the use of tampons may be a co-factor, somewhat increasing the odds of a TSS episode. If the offending bacteria/viruses are already present and the patient's vulnerability is high . . . the use of a tampon could conceivably increase the risk."

Although Edwards proceeded to outline several steps P&G should take in light of the CDC briefing, none included

sharing with P&G customers or the public the information
P&G had learned about the link between tampons and TSS.
He rejected the idea of abandoning the production and sales
of tampons and called for a vigorous defense of Rely in the
public relations area. Since sanitary napkins were not linked
to TSS, Edwards suggested reevaluating P&G's decision not
to get into sanitary napkins. He recommended P&G prepare
for "expected questions from the press, stock analysts, customers and consumerists."

P&G prepared a question and answer form for its sales force
in case they were asked about tampons and TSS. The form
contained misinformation and half truths as to what
P&G knew about tampons and Toxic Shock Syndrome. In
response to the question: "Are you aware that Toxic Shock
Syndrome has been associated with tampon use?" the answer
P&G told its sales people to give was:

> "In most of the cases surveyed, there has been a high level
> of tampon use but the CDC has indicated that it is very
> unlikely that tampon use causes the disease."

P&G's prepared response to the question did not disclose
the existence of the CDC study linking tampons to TSS in
menstruating women. The statement that "most of the cases
surveyed" had a "high level of tampon use" was understated,
given the fact that the level in the CDC study was 100 percent,
and in the Wisconsin study it was 97 percent. But the most
serious misinformation was contained in the statement regarding the CDC. The CDC stated in the *MMWR* of June 27,
1980, that tampon use *by itself* is not sufficient to cause the
disease. That is a far cry from saying that it is "very unlikely
that tampon use causes the disease." Moreover, the *MMWR*
proposed that the tampon might act as a cofactor and that the
use of tampons might favor growth of the *Staphylococcus aureus*
bacterium in the vagina.

Throughout the summer of 1980, P&G remained silent about
tampons and TSS, and it continued to promote aggressively
the sale of Rely tampons. In July, it mailed free samples to

two million households, and it maintained its radio and television advertising campaign. On June 27, 1980, the day the CDC published its *MMWR* report on tampons and Toxic Shock Syndrome, Kathryn Kehm, daughter of Michael and Pat Kehm of Cedar Rapids, Iowa, was twenty-seven days old. She and her two-year-old sister, Andrea, would know their mother only seventy-one more days—because the box of Rely tampons Pat bought in late August and used in early September did not warn her about TSS or tell her what to do if the symptoms appeared. No box of Rely would ever carry such a warning.

P&G not only knew from the CDC about the TSS association with tampons but was aware of the advisability of removing the tampon immediately upon the first signs of TSS. Bruce Dan of the CDC had told P&G and the other tampon manufacturers about the importance of this following the completion of the CDC study. P&G's Owen Carter, who was at the Atlanta briefing, admitted that his company knew early in the summer of 1980 about the necessity of removing the tampon immediately upon the signs and symptoms of TSS. And, as soon as the CDC report was released in the June 27, 1980 *MMWR*, Dr. Todd would tell anyone who asked that the tampon should be removed upon the appearance of the first signs of TSS. But it would not be until August 27, 1980—six days before Pat Kehm would begin using Rely tampons for the first time in her life—that P&G contacted Todd, even though he was then considered the leading authority on TSS.

The P&G attitude about tampons and TSS during the summer of 1980 may be reflected best by the reaction of company official Dale Haverstadt after he was informed that the government claimed that tampons helped cause TSS: "Next it will be Pampers!"

While Pat Kehm was dying of Toxic Shock Syndrome, the CDC began its second retrospective case control study of TSS in menstruating women. Unlike the first CDC study (CDC I), this study would be able to examine brand differences because there were enough new TSS cases in July and August to constitute an adequate sample. The "index period" would be the same for both cases and controls. The young CDC doctors would be comparing use of tampon brands by cases and controls during the same time frame. They were anxious to see if their study would single out any particular component of a tampon for the alarming TSS epidemic that health officials were witnessing in America. As the data were being collected and fed into the CDC computer, an unmistakable trend was emerging. The revolutionary new tampon that had not even been available in all parts of the United States until a few months before was showing a disproportionately high involvement in TSS cases. Later, Bruce Dan wrote a personal account of the CDC's hectic efforts to release their second study:

"We . . . started collecting cases during July and August and by the end of August had almost 50 cases which with the planned 150 controls would give us a statistically valid study. . . .

It was an incredible task to try and contact 50 women all over the country when all we really had was their name, the city or town they were hospitalized in (which might not correspond to their hometowns), and their doctor's name.

Since it was a holiday weekend [Labor Day] we were virtually alone in the CDC, staying up twenty hours a day and trying to make calls. . . .

By Monday morning most, but not all, of the data were collected and they were being entered into a computer . . . . We were all hand-tallying the data and obviously were seeing the trend. We knew by Tuesday morning what the answer would be: do we wait for the computer and statistical calculations that would verify it and pass it by peer review both inside and outside the Center so we would be sure of the data, or do we get it out in the *MMWR* that next week because women were dying?

After agonizing discussions with our chiefs (John Bennett, head of the Bacterial Diseases Division, and Foege) we decided that in order to make a pronouncement of this magnitude we had better be sure."

On September 13, 1980, seven days after Pat's death from TSS, the CDC completed its second study of fifty TSS cases. As Shands, Dan and the other doctors went over the data, they realized that a major part of the TSS mystery appeared to be solved. Seventy-one percent of the victims were using one brand of tampons while only 26 percent of the control group used that tampon—Procter & Gamble's Rely. The task-force doctors rechecked and verified their computations and then wasted no further time in reporting their findings to Dr. William Foege, director of the CDC and assistant surgeon general of the United States. Foege immediately passed the information on to Paul Hile of the FDA's Office of Regulatory Affairs.

When Hile examined the results of the second CDC study, he knew the FDA had no choice but to act. P&G was immediately briefed on the second CDC study and summoned to a meeting at the FDA in Washington, D.C., on September 16, 1980, to discuss its ramifications. A delegation of thirteen P&G executives, headed by Thomas Laco, executive vice president, and Powell McHenry, vice president and general counsel, left Cincinnati in a company jet to attend the meeting. They brought with them a proposed TSS warning to be printed on boxes of Rely tampons that they hoped would satisfy the FDA.

Representing the CDC at the meeting were Shands, Dan and Dr. George Schmid, a fellow EIS officer who was a member of the TSS task force at the CDC. The FDA had twelve officials attend, including Hile and Nancy Buc, a young and relatively inexperienced FDA lawyer.

After everyone had been introduced, Hile told the P&G officials of the "FDA's grave concern about Rely's heavier association with TSS." He said it "presented a significant and unusual risk to users," and he told P&G that "we feel Rely should be removed from the market and that users should be notified of the risks involved in the use of this device."

The P&G officials objected, and they advised the FDA of a P&G public opinion study that showed that only 20 percent of American women had heard of TSS compared to 71 percent of California women. They argued that there was considerable news coverage in California of TSS and that this had increased public awareness in California about TSS in general and, since Rely was often mentioned, about the P&G brand of tampons in particular. They contended that the just-completed second CDC study may have been biased by the news coverage.

Dan responded by pointing out that a high percentage of the TSS cases in CDC I, the June 1980 study, also showed Rely brand association. A P&G official then argued that even the first study was conducted "at a time of high publicity which could have impact on the results obtained." Dan retorted that the news linking tampons to TSS did not appear until after CDC I had been completed.

When P&G pressed its claim that publicity about Rely could have affected the validity of both CDC studies, FDA lawyer Buc pointed out:

> "If publicity has had an effect on CDC results, it seems logical it would be reflected in the controls as well as the subjects, which is not the case."

As a compromise, P&G's delegation offered to enter into an educational program for consumers and physicians after it held a Scientific Advisory Group conference. They told the FDA that the conference intended to examine what course of action and further studies with respect to Rely were indicated.

The FDA recessed the meeting for an hour, and when they reconvened, Hile told P&G to review the CDC data and then:

> "Inform us why you believe a recall of Rely is not appropriate."

Hile told the P&G officials that the FDA would draft a press release about CDC II and that the CDC would release the study the next day in the *MMWR*. At that point, members of the P&G group became extremely agitated, and they asked the FDA to suppress any specific reference to Rely in the release of the CDC study, pointing out that such publicity "would cause irreparable damage to Rely in the marketplace." FDA lawyer Buc pointedly turned down P&G's request, stating that Rely would be publicly mentioned because it was part of the study. She added that it would be wrong for the FDA not to do so.

The meeting ended with the understanding that the FDA would give P&G a short time to prove why a recall should not be ordered. It was informally agreed that they would reconvene in one week. The next morning P&G executives flew down to Atlanta to persuade Dr. Foege against releasing the results of CDC II. According to Bruce Dan:

> "Foege of course said he couldn't withhold that sort of information from the public. They then suggested that he just omit any reference to the specific name of the product. Foege said no dice. They then left and flew directly to Washington to meet with Pat Harris [Secretary of Health] in an attempt to go over Foege's head. She wouldn't meet with them. They then went to see Ohio Congressmen . . ."

The following day, September 17, 1980, the CDC publicly released the results of its second study on Toxic Shock Syndrome, and the announcement received extensive news media coverage. P&G's toll free phone became swamped with callers. Its consumer service officials answered the callers by calmly reading a press release that said "TSS is very rare" and it "isn't carried by tampons." When callers asked what the company's recommendation about Rely was, the P&G spokesman would respond:

> "The bottom line is that it's really a personal decision as to what you want to do."

In a prepared statement released to the news media, P&G protested that the CDC information was "too limited and fragmentary for any conclusions to be drawn." P&G also claimed it had thoroughly tested the safety of Rely before introducing the product and added:

> "In all of the extensive testing and use by millions of women, we have never found any evidence of a serious illness caused by this product."

Two days later, on September 19, 1980, a reporter discovered that P&G had quietly stopped production of Rely tampons at its manufacturing plants. When questioned about this, a P&G spokesman optimistically predicted that the shutdown would be short in duration and that production would resume after the CDC study results had been properly analyzed.

Simultaneously, P&G began its defense of Rely by claiming the findings might have been biased:

> "Earlier publicity about this disease is likely to have increased complaints forwarded to the Center and the CDC got caught up in the avalanche of publicity."

This criticism would become more sophisticated after P&G hired three Yale doctors to look for flaws in the two CDC studies. P&G had not been impressed with the logic of FDA lawyer Buc that if the TSS cases had been influenced by publicity to name Rely as the brand they were using, the same publicity effect should have been seen in the controls.

On September 19, 1980, Utah released the results of its expanded study, which showed the same high involvement of Rely as CDC II. With that development, the FDA asked Procter & Gamble to move up the date for its next joint meeting to Tuesday, September 23, 1980.

On Sunday, September 21, 1980, P&G held a hastily called meeting at Chicago's O'Hare Hilton of scientists it called the Scientific Advisory Group. The group consisted of five scientists, three of whom were physicians who had received compensation from P&G for past consulting services. They included Tommy Evans, the gynecologist from Wayne State University who had been on the first Rely Scientific Advisory Group, which had given its seal of approval to the safety testing for Rely. The two scientists present who had not previously been P&G consultants were James Todd of Denver and Patrick Schlievert, Rudolph Galask's "star protégé."

Prior to the meeting, P&G had mailed the group a summary of information on TSS and tampon usage. The five scientists made a significant change in the conclusion entitled "Current Assessments." P&G had proposed the scientists endorse the assertion that:

> "It is clearly the consensus of all investigators studying TSS that tampons are not the cause of TSS."

However, all five scientists refused to approve that statement and insisted that it be amended by insertion of the word *sole* to read:

> "It is clearly the consensus of all investigators studying TSS that tampons are not the sole cause of TSS."

The scientists also advised P&G that the CDC and state health department studies could not be ignored and that there was no scientific defense to the FDA's request for a recall.

The following day, September 22, 1980, Edward Harness, then P&G chairman of the board, who had rushed back to Cincinnati from a meeting with Japanese business interests on the West Coast, convened a meeting of top P&G officials. Harness, whose entire background was in advertising and who lacked any scientific expertise, found his office crowded with P&G personnel. He asked that most of the people present leave, stating: "I don't know how to make a decision in a ball park," and then asked those who remained their opinion on whether P&G should ride out the storm or pull the product off the market. Harness found three arguments for pulling the product particularly persuasive. First, that the product could not survive the bad publicity anyway—P&G's marketing department had reported that a *de facto* recall was already happening.

"Supermarket chains and discount houses, like Safeway,
Giant, Woolworth, National and Grand Union, have taken
the product off the shelves. They won't sell it and its
bound to spread. It's dead, anyway."

The second argument was that the FDA would require a
recall—and it could be voluntary or involuntary. P&G's legal
counsel expressed a preference for the voluntary route since a
recall would be admissible in evidence against P&G in the
inevitable products liability suits that would be filed. The third
argument was that the continuing controversy over Rely could
have an adverse fall-out effect on other P&G products.

After hearing the arguments, Harness told them that he was
in favor of the preemptive strike—beating the FDA to the
punch. He polled each of the other key executives to see if
they agreed with the decision. It was unanimous. That afternoon, one day before it was to meet with the FDA, P&G
announced that it was voluntarily suspending the sale of Rely.

The following day, September 23, 1980, Hile told P&G
officials that his agency was contemplating invoking federal
law to compel P&G to engage in a notification and retrieval/
refund program—a recall of Rely. P&G officials responded
by formally advising the FDA that it had suspended the sale
of Rely tampons and would ask that customers send the product to Cincinnati for a refund. FDA lawyer Buc told the
P&G officials that that was not good enough. She insisted
that there be a formal consent agreement spelling out P&G's
obligations, which included conducting a comprehensive advertising program to ensure that all Rely tampon users were
informed and a requirement that neither Rely, nor a product
identical to it, be reintroduced to the marketplace without prior
FDA approval. At first P&G objected to a consent agreement,
and several hours elapsed before they consented to such a settlement and its terms.

Three days later, on September 26, 1980, Procter & Gamble signed the consent agreement. It provided, among other
things, that (1) P&G would discontinue all sales of Rely, (2)

P&G would make every reasonable effort to withdraw any advertisement for Rely placed prior to September 22, 1980, (3) P&G would conduct a consumer notification and retrieval program especially designed to reach the eighteen to thirty-four-year-old group of women, and (4) P&G could not reintroduce Rely tampons without the prior written permission of the FDA.

FDA commissioner Jere E. Goyan was proud of his agency's action in the tampon controversy. Speaking in Washington, D.C., on October 2, 1980, to a tampon manufacturers trade group called the Health Industry Manufacturers Association, of which Procter & Gamble was a member, Goyan also lauded Procter & Gamble.

Apparently unaware of what went on at the FDA meetings with P&G, he claimed that the company had acted on its own initiative in recalling Rely. He also asserted that publicity surrounding the CDC II study had resulted in a number of lawsuits against P&G. Actually, P&G had been sued once (a California case in August 1980) before CDC II had even commenced, and there were only two lawsuits between the release of CDC II and before Goyan spoke to the trade group. In addition, Goyan said P&G had acted responsibly and in the public interest in agreeing to the consent agreement plan. Families of TSS death victims who died in the summer of 1980 saw it differently—P&G's action came far too late and was hardly responsible.

P&G exploited Goyan's benevolence. The company's public relations department transformed the act of staying one step ahead of the law into an act of martyrdom. The claim of "voluntary action" was repeatedly emphasized. The public announcements required by the FDA in the consent agreement repeated the myth on television, over the radio and in the printed media. Press kits distributed by P&G's public relations department on the eve of Rely toxic shock trials would emphasize the voluntary nature of the recall in an effort to influence a favorable jury decision by generating public opinion support for P&G.

Even television personality Phil Donahue was so moved by P&G propaganda that he said about the forced withdrawal:

> "I think Procter & Gamble would want you to know—incidentally, a company that I thought exercised excellent corporate responsibility in this area. They lost a lot of money and I'm not asking for a standing ovation, but in an age of greed and diminishing profits not all companies have been as fast as I thought P&G was in this matter. I think P&G is sitting there silently and I think they are proud of the way they handled it too. I think they got the focus because they sold the most product. Rely was the highest selling item."

Donahue's lack of information is revealed by his statement that Rely was the highest selling item. It wasn't. Tampax enjoyed more than a 2 to 1 lead over P&G's Rely in sales. P&G merely expected to overtake Tampax someday. That may explain why P&G did not warn about TSS in the summer of 1980 while women and young girls were getting deathly sick, and in some cases dying, from Toxic Shock Syndrome as a result of using Rely and other tampons. But, as Frank N. Magid, an expert on television news research once observed: "It is not what things actually are, but what people perceive things to be that is important to them." Through relentless repetition of the claim that its action was voluntary, that is eventually what was perceived to be true.

Ironically, after Rely was removed from the marketplace, P&G's officials became advocates of tampon labeling about TSS. P&G officials filed briefs with the FDA in support of TSS warnings on tampon boxes, which, at that time, could only apply to their former tampon competitors.

P&G was looking to the future. When the company took Rely off the market, its vice president Edwards listed objectives to be accomplished at a meeting with the FDA. One was to "convince the CDC and the FDA they must establish standards of performance and labeling under which Rely, or other catamenial products, can enter the market." Whether P&G's

interest in requiring labeling was humanitarian or an effort to establish standards for P&G's reentry into the menstrual products market may have been answered by the fact that P&G began test marketing in Minneapolis and St. Paul a mini-pad called "Always"—about two years after the recall of Rely. But the recall of Rely had been costly to P&G. Its newest product, upon which the company had pinned such high hopes, had been destroyed in the marketplace, and P&G wrote off $75 million in anticipated losses associated with the development and promotion of Rely. However, P&G's withdrawal of Rely, painful as it was to the company and its stockholders, came too late to help Pat Kehm and the other American women who died during the summer and early fall of 1980.

Surveying the wreckage surrounding the Rely disaster and the anticipated claims of TSS victims, P&G had to decide: Should it apologize for what happened and pay fair compensation to the victims, or should it concede nothing and use its enormous resources to resist all claims, whether valid or not? Should P&G be contrite or fight?

TWO

P&G, Tampons and TSS

5

"I do not see anything in it which should give P&G any concern."

P&G-funded scientist reassuring P&G about his proposed manuscript.

P&G officials allowed themselves little time to commiserate over the loss of a promising new product and the research and development costs that would not be recaptured. Instead, their attention was focused on the anticipated wave of lawsuits for sickness or death from Rely tampons. The first such suit had been filed by Linda Imboden of Redding, California, on August 6, 1980—six weeks before the CDC II study would show Rely tampons increased the user's chance of getting TSS by threefold over other tampons. The California housewife sued for $5 million, claiming that she lost parts of her fingers and toes as a result of getting TSS from using Rely tampons.

By the end of October 1980, a half dozen more suits had been filed against P&G in connection with the recalled tampon; one of them was the suit filed by Mike Kehm. Several hundred more suits were being readied for filing as lawyers for victims or their survivors sought to learn about the strange new illness and its apparent connection with the seemingly innocuous tampon—a product that had been used by millions of women for more than forty years without serious illness or injury. By the time most of these suits would be filed, P&G was far advanced in the development and implementation of a carefully drawn strategy to deal with them. The strategy that P&G rejected was contrition. The strategy it adopted was denial, stonewalling and the legal, although morally questionable, suppression of evidence.

P&G's decision to stonewall was not without precedent. P&G resisted when environmentalists appealed for the removal of phosphates from detergents in order to slow down and reverse the pollution of American rivers and lakes. After public appeals failed and a handful of local governments began to pass ordinances against phosphates and detergents, P&G abandoned those markets rather than comply with the law. Its competition, Lever Brothers, chose to comply with the ordinances. It was only after several states passed laws banning phosphates that P&G complied. P&G's attitude was that it was not the company's responsibility to worry about pollution in the streams but that of local government to provide proper sewage treatment to remove the phosphates.

P&G's law firm for the TSS litigation was Dinsmore & Shohl, of Cincinnati. The company's ties to the sixty-plus member law firm were strengthened several years earlier when a senior partner, Powell McHenry, left the firm to become vice president and general counsel of Procter & Gamble. McHenry is a Harvard law school graduate whose soft-spoken and genteel manner hides a toughness that befits his job as top legal officer of one of the largest corporate conglomerates in the world. No major decision in TSS litigation would be implemented without McHenry's prior approval. The earliest, and most fundamental, decision made by P&G was to deny that Rely was in any way responsible for TSS. P&G opted to commit its vast wealth to fight claims of TSS victims rather than use a small part of its wealth to compensate the victims. The strategy P&G adopted would force TSS victims to settle for a fraction of the true value of their claims. The method would be to make TSS litigation so expensive the victims could not afford the high costs of going to court against P&G.

A multifaceted plan was approved in September 1980 by the Rely Litigation Group, which consisted of Dinsmore & Shohl attorneys and personnel from P&G assigned to assist in the defense of Rely TSS cases. The first and highest priority of the plan was to obtain the services of all scientists who were already working in the field of TSS research or who showed an interest in doing so.

The plan was simple. P&G would offer substantial financial grants to scientists who were studying TSS (a grant to one scientist exceeded, $400,000). But there were to be strings attached—an important one was the understanding that a scientist could not publish a report on his research without letting P&G review the manuscript in advance. P&G would get to see the results of the scientist's work twenty-one days before it could be submitted to any scientific journal for publication.

P&G did not try the approach that industry once found popular. A grant in the 1930s, for example, provided that any manuscript would be "submitted to Johns-Manville Company for approval prior to publication." Despite the absence of a similar proviso, P&G expected the same result with its funding of scientists as Johns-Manville had. It trusted that scientists would fulfill the company's expectations so as to remain in P&G's good graces when the time came to make a decision on renewing the large grant.

An example of the scientists' desire not to offend P&G is a memo from Dr. David Tamplin, of the University of Miami School of Medicine, to P&G. In connection with a proposed manuscript that he submitted to the company on March 1, 1983, Tamplin reassured P&G:

> "I do not see anything in it which should give P&G any concern."

Tamplin, who signed his letter as "Professor of Dermatology, Professor of Epidemiology and Public Health, and Chief

of the Division of International Community Medicine," asked
P&G if it would be all right not to let the reader know that
the research was financed by P&G because:

> "It would be a pity to think of the work as a 'drug com-
> pany' study."

The Rely Litigation Group apparently believed that by
making large grants it would be easy to nudge scientific inquiry gently into obscure research and away from areas that
might prove why tampons increase a menstruating woman's
chance of getting TSS. Tamplin's research, while dealing with
Toxic Shock Syndrome generally, did not address the question of the tampon role in TSS. And that was just the way
P&G wanted it.

As P&G anticipated, its program to corner the scientific
market in TSS met with immediate success. Faced with the
prospect of declining federal research grants as a conservative
administration was about to take power, scientists working in
TSS were eager to accept P&G's offers of funding. Only one
scientist—a microbiologist by the name of Tierno—would reject P&G's offers.

From the early fall of 1980, when P&G began its research
funding project, the company would proclaim that it was
funding research for the advancement of science and the good
of humanity. Three years later, P&G would refuse to divulge
the results of certain unfavorable research findings, claiming
that it was "privileged." Yet, it would admit that its financing
of scientists came from its Rely defense fund—the same fund
that paid its attorneys and all other defense costs in the TSS
litigation.

From the Rely Litigation Group's standpoint, it was a bar-
gain to invest in TSS research for the $3 million that P&G
would spend. The threat posed by a thousand or more lawsuits and the political liability for both compensatory and punitive damages was the reason.

Compensatory damages are damages awarded not to punish, as in the case of punitive damages, but to compensate a

victim for the loss that he or she has sustained. Compensatory damages include what are known as "special" damages, or "out-of-pocket expenses," such as loss of past and future income and past and future medical and hospital expense. Compensatory damages also include "general" damages, such as pain and suffering, partial or total disability, which reduces enjoyment of life, and, in death cases, loss of services, love and affection of a spouse and parent.

In all but four states, the law allows punitive damage awards to punish and deter a wrongdoer from conduct that is considered outrageous. The conduct must be more than mere negligence. It must be conduct so indifferent to the rights of others as to amount to a reckless or wanton disregard for human safety. The amount of a punitive damage award may be based on the net worth and income of the defendant. A Tennessee court put it succinctly: "What would be smart money to a poor man would not serve as a deterrent to a rich man."

In 1980, the year Pat Kehm died, P&G was worth about $5 billion and earned $643 million after taxes. A plaintiff's attorney suing P&G for a toxic shock illness or death could argue that if a drunk driver making $20,000 a year caused a similar injury or death, it would not be unthinkable to assess him with a punitive damage fine of $2,000, or 10 percent of his income. If the same argument were then applied to P&G's $643 million, the verdict would be $64 million in punitive damages. The attorney could argue that it would take the same percentage to "smart" either defendant because of the disparity in wealth. Conceivably, the jury might agree that $2000 taken from a man earning $20,000 a year would "smart" even more than taking $64 million from a corporation making $643 million.

Considering the number of cases that might be filed, $100 million in aggregate compensatory damages was not an unrealistic prospect should juries become antagonistic toward P&G's handling of the Toxic Shock Syndrome issue. But the potential for punitive damages was even greater should the juries find that P&G was reckless or wanton either in the design of Rely, in inadequate testing of it or in failing to warn the consumer after it knew about the tampon association with TSS. Therefore, P&G's decision to commit $3 million from its defense fund for scientific research in TSS was a well thought-out business decision—not the philanthropic act that P&G's public relations department would claim.

It was a shrewd decision because it would put P&G in a no-lose situation. At best, although improbable, P&G's funded research conceivably might show tampons were innocent of any role in TSS. That would justify many times the amount P&G committed to the research. At the very least, P&G would be viewed as humanitarian in its claimed "quest for scientific truth."

In between best and worst situations lay a number of advantages to P&G. The substantial infusion of research money would ingratiate P&G with the scientific community generally and with those grantees in particular, thereby creating a climate of goodwill that had limitless possibilities for benefit to P&G. Certainly, P&G could expect a grantee would be less harsh in his criticism should his research indict P&G. In addition, the grants gave P&G immediate access to TSS research. The world of scientific research moves slowly and the goal of a scientist is to be published. In some cases, his livelihood depends on it. To publish, a scientist must painstakingly check and recheck his testing data. Then, his manuscript is sent to a scientific journal for publication. But before accepting it, the journal sends the manuscript to two experts in the field for "peer review." All of this takes time.

By funding scientific research, P&G guaranteed itself immediate and limitless access to the scientific research on TSS—a tremendous advantage over its competitors as well as the victims of TSS. They would have to wait for its publication in a journal—publication that might never come. This would allow P&G to enter into settlement negotiations with victims who were in the dark as to any recent scientific evidence that would strengthen their case.

Moreover, P&G was also conducting its own in-house research. Access to the leading TSS scientists in the United States and abroad would permit P&G to have advantages that each of the scientists it funded, acting independently, would lack. In its in-house research, P&G would not have to reinvent the wheel but could build upon the information coming from the outside researchers.

Another advantage of the grants, in my view, was that they gave P&G the opportunity to suppress, or at least delay, the release of information hurtful to P&G. The advantages of delay in release of information were more important to P&G than to its tampon competitors because the "statute of limitations"—deadlines on the time an injured person can bring a lawsuit against the wrongdoer—could very well run out.

P&G recalled Rely from the marketplace in September of 1980, and virtually all claims would have been based on illness occurring before October 1, 1980. In most states, claims would be barred if they were not filed before October 1, 1982. By delaying release of damaging scientific research long enough, P&G would be beyond the period of suit. In addition, those cases that would have been filed within the allowable time period would have been tried or settled without the TSS victims' attorneys ever having the benefit of all the scientific information.

In accepting P&G money for research into TSS, the grant recipients created for themselves a clear conflict of interest. As independent scientists, they were taking money from a company that was interested in the results of their research—not from the standpoint of developing a new product or improving an existing product but to vindicate past conduct.

In most instances, P&G was able to suggest the subject of inquiry, and by directing scientific research into areas removed from the role that tampons play in TSS and into collateral inquiries, P&G was, in effect, side-lining research investigators from the central issue. An exception was Merlin Bergdoll, a researcher at the University of Wisconsin, who began his work on the tampon connection before receiving funding from P&G.

P&G funded both Davis of Wisconsin and Todd of Colorado to conduct active surveillance of TSS cases occurring after the recall of Rely. Surveillance prior to the recall had been passive. Active surveillance could be expected to turn up more cases of TSS than passive—like affirmative action in seeking out minorities to hire is more successful than a passive program. The CDC had reported a drop-off of TSS cases after the recall of Rely. P&G's objective in turning up more TSS cases after Rely had been recalled than would otherwise be counted would tend to show that Rely was innocent of causing TSS. At the same time, casting doubt on the CDC would serve to cast doubt on the CDC studies.

P&G found another way to cast doubt on the CDC studies. On December 2, 1980, Davis and his Minnesota counterpart, Michael Osterholm, were lectured by P&G advertising expert, M.D. Seymour. According to a P&G memo dated December 8, 1980: "A discussion given by Mr. Seymour on the 'recall' effect due to promotional advertising seemed to impress Osterholm and Davis and to let them really understand how Rely could have such a large apparent share of the TSS reported cases."

The lecture apparently had an effect. Davis published an article of re-interviews with TSS victims who had had their onset of illness prior to July 1, 1980. He found inconsistencies between some women's original response pertaining to tampon brands used during their illness and their response when interviewed after the publicity about the recall of Rely. He found that the inconsistencies usually reflected the additional reporting of Rely tampon usage. He implied that the CDC and other epidemiological studies may have been flawed by the fact that intense media publicity about Rely tampons influenced women to name Rely when they were actually using another brand at the time they became ill. He overlooked the fact that CDC I and his own Wisconsin study were carried out before there was any publicity about tampons and TSS and that the CDC

II study was carried out before there was any media publicity about Rely and TSS. In fact, it was the release of the completed CDC II study that generated the adverse publicity about Rely.

There were two additional benefits to P&G scientific funding. One was that the scientist might stumble upon a vaccine or a preventative for TSS or figure out how to make a safe tampon. If that occurred, P&G would have the competitive advantage needed to reenter the tampon market and swiftly overtake the present leader, Tampax. The other benefit was the fact that it could expect experts it had funded to show up as witnesses at TSS trials. It would be unlikely that a scientist like Todd, who could not be subpoenaed outside of Colorado, would travel thousands of miles to give testimony in cases in which he had no interest. A $403,000 grant might encourage such cooperation.

The second part of the Rely Litigation Group's strategy was a refinement of the old divide and conquer objective. In this case, P&G intended to keep the "enemy" divided before they could get together. In P&G's eyes, the enemy consisted of TSS victims and their lawyers. The method by which P&G would carry out its objective was a seldom used provision in the court rules for granting of "protective orders" to prevent the disclosure of trade secrets and similar confidential data.

The Rely Litigation Group knew that since TSS was a new phenomenon and its link to tampons murky and far from scientifically established, the attorneys of TSS victims would be in the dark about how to prove a TSS case against P&G. The Rely Litigation Group hoped to keep it that way. What they feared most was that attorneys for plaintiffs would mount a cooperative effort to exchange information uncovered in their individual lawsuits. If this were to happen, the TSS victims would be better prepared in court, and the cost of getting prepared would be spread around, making the litigation less expensive. The courts have long recognized that it makes no sense to force each attorney for victims with similar claims to have to repeat the discovery already uncovered by other plaintiffs. In a Colorado products liability lawsuit against Ford Motor Company, federal judge James Carrigan said it best:

> "To so require would be tantamount to holding that each litigant who wishes to ride a taxi to court must undertake the expense of inventing the wheel."

P&G did not subscribe to Judge Carrigan's rationale and applied to the courts for protective orders. Under those terms, when a TSS victim's lawyer filed a request to P&G to produce documents relating to Rely tampons, the company could legally refuse unless the lawyer signed an agreement that the documents would be shown only to witnesses in that particular case. These witnesses would also have to sign the agreement to keep the documents confidential. Even if plaintiffs' lawyers agreed to sign the protective order, P&G would not have to produce the requested documents in the city where the trial was to be held. Instead, P&G could insist that they travel to Cincinnati, Ohio, at their own expense and search through 600,000 P&G documents, many of which were duplicates, in the hope of finding information relevant to Rely tampons and TSS. As P&G correctly envisioned it, many plaintiffs' lawyers would give up and settle cheaply rather than spend the time and energy, not to mention the expense, of looking for a needle in such a large haystack. P&G also reasoned that those determined enough to make the trip to Ohio might easily miss finding what they were looking for. Even if a lawyer might stumble upon something helpful, that lawyer, alone, would have the information and could not share it with other lawyers representing TSS victims.

There was one more important benefit to P&G. Under ordinary circumstances, requested documents are marked and identified so that if the party required to deliver the documents would omit something, and it later turned up, the court could punish the party who held back the documents. Under P&G's procedure of allowing discovery, the company need not worry about anyone making such a claim because, in a collection of some 600,000 documents, who could say that the missing document was not there and was simply overlooked?

P&G's dual justification for a protective order was that there were far too many cases and documents to be shipped back and forth all over the country and that many of the documents contained P&G trade secrets and other proprietary information. P&G spared no document from the confidential designation—including published newspaper articles. Since Rely tampons had been taken off the market under a cloud of sickness and death that seemed to deny its ever being a viable product for P&G or anyone else, it was difficult to believe that Rely had valuable trade secrets worth protecting. Recognizing P&G's true motive, some lawyers for TSS victims would refuse to agree voluntarily to the terms of the proposed protective order. Although the argument about trade secrets was little more than a smokescreen, the courts in the TSS cases took the easiest path and granted P&G's request for a protective order. The alternative would have required the court to examine hundreds of documents—a time-consuming (and time-wasting) task. It may be that the judges decided it was more expedient to give P&G what it wanted than to require every court in which a TSS claim had been filed to pass on the confidentiality of so many documents.

Assuming, perhaps, that research connecting tampons to TSS would either not be developed or, if it were, would not be released, P&G's final strategy was to undermine the only case that TSS victims had—the circumstantial evidence provided by the epidemiological studies. They accomplished this by hiring the nation's leading authority on epidemiological studies, Dr. Alvan Feinstein, of Yale University. With the aid of his two colleagues, Ralph Horowitz and Mary Harvey, Feinstein prepared a detailed analysis of every criticism that could be theoretically raised about the manner in which the CDC I and CDC II studies were carried out. Their bottom-line conclusion, which they promised P&G they would testify to in court, was that the epidemiological studies by the CDC and the state public health departments were invalid.

Having positioned itself to control laboratory evidence of the Rely connection to TSS and having employed the best experts to deal with the only evidence available—the circumstantial proof of the epidemiological studies—P&G was now ready to go to court to take on the victims of TSS or their families who blamed Rely tampons for the injuries or deaths.

6

"Imagine hundreds of . . . 'toxin factories' or 'toxin chambers' in every super absorbent tampon. The super absorbency of the product brings in enormous amounts of nutrients to insure this phenomenon."

Dr. Philip M. Tierno, Jr.,
in his "open letter to Procter & Gamble,"
October 10, 1980.

I had hired my son, Peter, and his classmate, Todd Becker, in June of 1980, shortly after their graduation from law school. The new firm's offices, which were still under construction that summer, were a few hundred feet from the cemetery where Pat Kehm would lay buried. As members of my new firm, Peter and Todd were unable to work in the old firm I would soon be leaving. The owner of the cemetery had just opened a new funeral home, so part of the old one was available for rent. While I was working downtown, Peter and Todd set up temporary offices at Cedar Memorial. They found a source of grim humor in having to occupy the former coffin room in their temporary quarters.

In September, my twenty-year-old daughter, Sara, a pre-law student, was hired as our new firm's receptionist. My secretary, Michele Askren, was promoted to legal assistant and was assigned to the Kehm file.

From time to time, the four of us, myself, Peter, Todd and Michele, would meet to discuss the case. In one of our earliest conferences, I told everyone that we were not only going to have to prove that Rely tampons caused Pat Kehm to have TSS but that Rely tampons can cause Toxic Shock Syndrome per se. We discussed P&G's reactions to the Kehm suit thus far; the company had filed an answer to the lawsuit denying that Rely had anything to do with TSS as well as denying that Pat died of the disease, and they had had plenty of opportunity to apologize or express regrets to their victims and had not. I reminded my staff of an old Persian saying: "Next to innocence, contrition is the best defense." P&G was not being contrite, so I concluded they intended to use innocence as a defense.

Peter volunteered that if P&G wanted to wage war they would not lack the means. He had seen a recent financial statement for the company that showed they had made $643 million in profits after taxes. I told him all the money in the world shouldn't change the fact that Pat Kehm used Rely for the first time on September 2, 1980, and four days later, she was dead.

Todd suggested that my comment was not a bad way to begin an opening statement to the jury. "I don't think so either," I said. "Yet, if Pat had been struck by a car four days later, we couldn't blame the tampon she was using, so we're still going to have to show a scientific connection and that means we're going to have to find an expert who can explain it or who, at least, has a credible theory for it."

I said I planned to contact the man who discovered Toxic Shock Syndrome. At the time, I couldn't think of anyone who would be more impressive. Naturally, I was unaware that Todd had already accepted a grant of $403,000 from P&G.

A lawsuit consists of five stages: preparing and filing the suit papers, conducting discovery, final trial preparation, the trial itself and an appeal. We were at the discovery stage.

When lawyers speak of discovery, they mean those procedures that let both sides of a lawsuit get testimony and documents from one another as well as from outsiders like witnesses unconnected with either party. One side can serve the other with written questions, called interrogatories, to be answered within a specific time, usually thirty days. Or, one side may take a deposition of the other or of an outside witness. At a deposition, the person answering the questions—the deponent—must answer under oath. A third common method of discovery is document production. One side must furnish the other with requested documents if he or she has them or is able to get them. A fourth method is to file a request for admissions in which the other side must admit or deny certain specific facts. In a major case, such as the Kehm case, all four methods of discovery are usually employed.

When suit was filed, I had named the Procter & Gamble Manufacturing Company and the Procter & Gamble Distributing Company as defendants. We had obtained those names from the Iowa Secretary of State's office registry of out of state corporations registered to do business in Iowa. It turned out they were both subsidiaries of P & G. After valuable time had been wasted, I learned that the tampons were manufactured by another subsidiary, P & G Paper Products Company—not the P & G Manufacturing Company. So, I filed an amendment to the suit papers bringing in the other subsidiary and the parent company as well. P & G's attorneys had not voluntarily disclosed that we had sued the wrong subsidiary. They waited the full length of time to answer interrogatories, in order to delay the litigation.

After the parent and the other subsidiary were in the lawsuit, we filed interrogatories to be answered by them. I also filed a request that P & G supply documents covering a number of subjects, including the design, manufacture and testing of Rely tampons, consumer complaints about Rely tampons and activities of P & G officials between CDC I and the recall of Rely.

Implementing its strategy not to provide information to a plaintiff's lawyer that could be exchanged with other plaintiffs' lawyers, P&G refused to produce any documents without a voluntary agreement by us for a protective order. Recognizing the maneuver by P&G for what it was, I refused and an impasse ensued.

It was momentarily broken when P&G attorneys took the deposition of Mike Kehm in April of 1981. The P&G attorney in charge of the deposition was Frank C. Woodside III, a medical doctor as well as an attorney. P&G capitalized on Mike Kehm's natural desire to avoid the limelight of courtroom involvement by asking sexual questions that were designed to embarrass and intimidate him.

> "In the months following the birth of your second child and Pat's death in September [three months later] did she have sexual intercourse with anybody other than you?"
>
> "No."

The company had not stopped with taking Pat Kehm's life. They degraded her memory and insulted her husband as well.

Reading the deposition, I was certain that P&G asked these types of questions to intimidate Mike Kehm into dropping his suit against P&G or, at the very least, to settle for a nominal amount. Later, in talking with other TSS victims, I learned that P&G often employed these tactics. This harassment worked in many cases. One young woman from South Dakota who had come close to dying from TSS as a result of using Rely tampons settled her claim for $15,000 because, as her mother told me: "She doesn't know if she can handle the insults and the intimate sexual questions at trial that had been asked at her deposition." A middle-aged TSS Rely victim from Iowa said that P&G deposition questions made her feel "cheap and dirty," yet her personal conduct had been exemplary.

The complaints of TSS victims about depositions taken by P&G were reminiscent of those voiced by rape victims after interrogations by insensitive policemen—that they, the victims, were somehow responsible for what had happened, and that they were the criminals instead of the victims.

As late as June 2, 1983, P&G was still engaged in the same tactics. A young North Carolina housewife had incurred TSS several months before her marriage in the fall of 1980. P&G wanted to know if she was having sex with her fiancé or anyone else at the time she got TSS. I had been called into the case to help the local attorney who represented her, and I decided to put an end to such irrelevant and harassing questions. Without knowing what her answer would be, I objected and instructed her not to answer the question. At a recess, I learned that this particular young lady was a virgin until her wedding night, something P&G market studies had probably predicted was against the law of averages. The young lady from North Carolina was neither proud nor ashamed of her virgin status at the time of her marriage but looked upon it as simply a fact. But it had nothing to do with TSS.

P&G's motives in asking such questions can be inferred from a 1982 deposition of an Iowa TSS victim who survived. Her lawyer objected and instructed the client not to answer sex-oriented questions unless P&G could show, by reference to scientific literature, that the answers to such questions had anything to do with TSS. Company attorneys threatened to seek a court order compelling the answer but never did so. If P&G had a genuine scientific interest in the answers to these types of questions, the company should have filed a motion to compel answers. It would appear P&G merely wanted to pose the questions, and it hoped that the victim, like the woman from South Dakota, would settle cheaply out of court. In the case of Mike Kehm, its tactic backfired. It only succeeded in making him angrier and more determined to fight P&G all the way.

During the impasse over the protective order, the *Chicago Tribune* ran an excellent seven-part series on tampons and toxic shock. From it I learned that the inventor of Tampax was still alive. A picture of the ninety-six-year-old osteopathic physician, Earl Haas, accompanied the story. It showed a spry man

with a few sprigs of hair on either side of his head. It said he
lived in Denver. I told Michele it was an interesting coincidence that the inventor of tampons and the man who discovered Toxic Shock Syndrome both lived in the same city.

After putting down the *Tribune*'s story, I contacted Dr. Haas
by telephone. The doctor said he was aware of the story but
had not seen it. I promised to send him a copy. Haas agreed
to give a deposition about the invention of the original tampax
and his opinion about its safety compared to the new superabsorbent tampons. I had not been able to get through to Todd
by telephone but thought that a personal visit to his office
would be difficult to rebuff. I was still not yet aware of Todd's
employment by P&G.

Nor did I know that the *Chicago Tribune* reporters had already been a target of attempted manipulation and evasion by
P&G in connection with the series on tampons and TSS. I
would eventually discover an April 3, 1981, P&G memo describing a meeting with Charlie Madigan of the Chicago Tribune News Service.

The memo stated that "Madigan was appreciative of the
information P&G provided to him" and that "he did not press
us on those areas we chose to avoid. For the most part, we
ignored his questionnaire."

Had I known about the memo before the Kehm trial, I would
have tried to find out what areas P&G chose to avoid and what
part of the *Tribune* questionnaire was ignored.

In June, my wife, Nan, and I went west, partly to relax at
a condominium we have at Lake Dillon in the heart of Colorado's ski country. On the second of that month, we visited
Dr. Haas. Haas's daughter was taking care of her father, who
was nearly blind and generally confined to bed. Despite this,
I found Haas's mind to be alert and his recall vivid. At one
point, he pointed proudly to a certificate on the wall that at-
tested to his still-current status as a licensed physician in Colorado.

Haas told how he had come to invent the tampon and that
he had been unsuccessful in interesting a manufacturing firm

to buy it. Haas had a stockbroker friend who he described as "quite an adept young fellow" who Haas sent "back East to contact some manufacturers back there, and all they gave him was the brush-off and he came home without anything. He talked to Johnson & Johnson and they said 'well, that will never sell in the world, and we wouldn't be interested in it at all' so he came home without anything."

Johnson & Johnson later changed its mind about tampons, but instead of enjoying the leadership role in the tampon market as owner of Tampax, it had to settle for next to last place in the tampon market with the product that it sold under the trade name of Meds. Later, Johnson & Johnson would drop Meds and introduce in its place a tampon called o.b.—a name not intended to connect it with the type of doctor who delivers babies but derived from the German *ohne binde*, which means "without napkin."

Haas did express the opinion that tampons should not block the vaginal vault. Since P&G admitted that Rely blocked the vagina, I felt that Haas's opinion would be of some weight to the jury. The way Haas put it seemed convincing:

> "I don't think that nature ever thought that flow should be stopped up see, and prohibited from coming out."

While I found Haas colorful, I realized that his testimony would be of limited value because Haas admitted knowing nothing about either superabsorbent tampons or Toxic Shock Syndrome.

I hoped to learn more about the disease when I stopped by the Children's Hospital of Denver where Dr. Todd had his offices. Arriving at the hospital, located in a dilapidated residential neighborhood just east of Denver's downtown area, I was told that Todd would not see lawyers for TSS victims except in conjunction with the taking of his deposition with P&G attorneys present. The charge that TSS victims would have to pay for learning Todd's views on TSS was $250 per hour, including the time that he would spend reading the transcript to see if there were any changes he wished to make.

I was shocked by a scientist's unwillingness to discuss a subject he had publicly written about. In twenty-five years of practicing law I had never encountered this attitude. I figured it would cost the typical TSS victim a couple of thousand dollars, including court reporter service and transportation expenses, just to find out if Todd had anything worthwhile to say about tampons and TSS—a lot of money for what we say in Iowa is "buying a pig in the poke." Disappointed that I was no further along in finding the explanation for the tampon and TSS connection, Nan and I started back for the mountains. Before leaving Denver, I called my office to check on messages. I was told that Steve Kaufman, a Denver lawyer, wanted to get together to discuss TSS.

Kaufman, who had gotten my name from Haas, was representing a young woman who had survived TSS. Kaufman told me he was interested in mounting a common effort to investigate the Rely connection and prepare for trial.

I said I would be up in the mountains for a couple days but agreed to meet with Kaufman before we returned to the Midwest.

My depression over the virtually wasted time spent in taking Haas's deposition and trying to meet Todd deepened as I made my way through documents obtained from Ralph Nader's Health Research Group. A memo from an FDA official by the name of Lillian Yin, who apparently had some responsibility with the FDA's Bureau of Medical Devices, did nothing to lighten my mood. Yin, in July 1980, had criticized CDC I as being premature on the basis of insufficient data connecting tampons to Toxic Shock Syndrome. That's just great, I thought. Here is an FDA bureaucrat, who's supposed to be protecting the lives of American women, and she is concerned about a government report being premature because she thinks the sample is too small. Instead of sounding the alarm so that the message would get out in July 1980, and lives like Pat Kehm's would be saved, Yin, it appeared, was siding with the tampon manufacturers. Even P&G didn't quarrel with the sample size, nor would its expert on such studies, Feinstein of Yale.

Whether Yin was right or wrong, I realized, P&G would seize upon that memo as justification for its continued promotion of Rely and its failure to warn during the summer of 1980. I was about to consider the day a total loss when I came across an "open letter" from a Philip Tierno, Ph.D., of Norwood, New Jersey, to P&G. He had sent a copy to the FDA, which the Nader group had obtained under the Freedom of Information Act. The letter was four pages long, and in it Tierno, a clinical microbiologist then at Goldwater Memorial Hospital of New York University Medical Center, explained how he had been asked by his wife why, as a user of superabsorbent tampons, she had not gotten TSS. After pointing out that a culture of his wife showed she did not have *Staph aureus* present, Tierno then proceeded to set out a fairly detailed hypothesis about how Rely tampons caused TSS. I had to read the letter over because I didn't understand much of the scientific jargon, but I liked Tierno's reference to Rely's synthetic particles as "hundreds of little toxin factories." I had no science courses in college, save for a fairly useless one in geology. My knowledge of pH was limited to hearing my wife say that she had to add some chemicals to the backyard swimming pool because the pH was getting too high or too low.

Yet, I recognized that it was not critical whether I understood or agreed with the Tierno theory—it was only important to have a scientific theory from an expert that the jury could hang its hat on if it wanted to compensate Mike Kehm and his two small daughters for the loss of a wife and mother. I told Nan that we might have found an expert—assuming that P&G hadn't offered him a grant, too.

The building in which the Denver lawyers had their offices was, like mine, several miles from the downtown area where the prestigious law firms are located.

It turned out the Denver lawyer was as inexperienced as my two associates, Peter and Todd, having also graduated from law school a year earlier. Tall, thin and with dark eyes and features, he sported a Sigmund Freud style beard and mustache—a distinct contrast to his boss, Jon Kidneigh, who struck me as the perfect role model of the public's conception of a laid-back Colorado ski instructor. His sandy light hair and tanned face matched up well with his casual western clothes.

I met first with Kaufman in his cramped office while Kidneigh was on the telephone. I listened as Kaufman told me of his client, Deletha Lampshire from Littleton, Colorado, an eighteen-year-old high school student at the time of her illness in May 1980. After six days in the hospital, she had recovered, and P&G was claiming that she had not had TSS and that her rash had probably been a result of a reaction to the antibiotic, ampicillin.

It turned out Kaufman had also obtained the Nader group material and I asked him what he thought of the Tierno letter. "It doesn't make sense," Kaufman replied. "I don't see why the white blood cells can't get in to attack the staph if the toxin is able to get out of those little toxin factories."

At that point, the secretary interrupted to say that Kidneigh was off the telephone, and we left Kaufman's small office for Kidneigh's more spacious one.

I told Kidneigh that Kaufman didn't think Tierno's theory made much sense. I went on to propose that it didn't matter whether Tierno was right or not. "He's got the necessary credentials to qualify as an expert, and I feel the jury will want to find for my client and his two kids if we can give them any scientific explanation that Rely causes TSS—whatever the scientific argument is and whether it's right or not." The clincher, I argued, was that: "You know and I know that Rely causes TSS. What is P&G going to do about Tierno's theory? The only way they can prove Tierno's theory is wrong is by proving what is right and that will still be that Rely tampons cause TSS. Besides, we don't have any choice because P&G has got everybody else in their hip pocket."

Kidneigh told Kaufman to get in touch with Tierno and find out if he was willing to go up against P&G and its team of experts. The meeting ended with the three of us agreeing to keep in touch and to share whatever information developed.

Back in Cedar Rapids, I called Tierno and told him that I had read the open letter to P&G and found it fascinating and insightful. I did not tell Tierno that I had failed to comprehend most of the scientific reasoning behind it. Tierno sounded pleased by my interest and said that he hadn't done any further work on tampons and TSS since writing the letter to P&G the previous fall. I asked if Tierno had received a response from P&G to the open letter. He told me that he had:

"The letter had gotten shuffled around at P&G and the same day it reached this fellow at P&G in Ohio, I got a call from him. He said he wanted to come right out and talk to me. I said we could talk over the telephone but he said that he was going to be in town anyway and wanted to talk about my theory. I had the feeling they were trying to buy me.

"They told me that they didn't believe my theory was possible, but that if I would apply for a P&G grant they would leave no stone unturned to see that I got every consideration," Tierno continued.

"It was strange the way they showed up at my office—they knew everything about me before they arrived, what I did, where I did it, where I had studied, what I had published and so on. It was eerie."

I could not help but remember what had happened in Rochester, New York, when the *Rochester Democrat and Chronicle* carried articles about consumer complaints concerning Procter & Gamble's Bounce fabric softener. After the first article appeared, the reporter got a call from P&G representatives asking her if they could "come out from Cincinnati and talk it over." According to the August 11, 1976, issue of the *Rochester Patriot*, the reporter said "no thanks," but P&G representatives nonetheless sought the reporter out in her newsroom. They explained, just as Tierno was told, that they "happened to be in the neighborhood and dropped in anyway." P&G, one of the nation's largest newspaper advertisers, asked the reporter not to publish a story on local dermatologists' opinions about possible Bounce-related skin reactions. The newspaper printed the article anyway.

I asked Tierno if he had changed his mind about the theory he had set out in his open letter of October 10, 1980. Tierno told me that there was no doubt but that Rely tampons were toxin factories.

When I asked how only a relatively few women got the disease, Tierno explained that there were several reasons. First, not every woman carried *Staph aureus* in her vagina flora and second, not all strains of *Staph* produce the toxin. Third, most women have been exposed to the toxin or some similar protein antigen in the past and have built up immunity to it.

I asked Tierno if he'd testify to that in court.

"I will if they don't get a contract out on me first," he replied half-seriously.

Tierno was obviously apprehensive for his safety since he was the only scientist willing to take on P&G. But he said he was willing to give a deposition. In some ways, he felt having his theory down on paper would put him out of danger.

In reporting to Kaufman about my talk with Tierno, I learned that Kidneigh and Kaufman were scheduled to take the depositions of eight P&G executives in Cincinnati on June 22 and 23, 1981. I asked if Kidneigh and Kaufman had any objection to my sitting in.

In order to participate in the depositions, I served a notice to do so to P&G. As soon as their attorneys got it, they went to federal court in Cedar Rapids to block my participation. Federal magistrate James Hodges, who was in charge of such pretrial matters, overruled P&G's objections with the comment that he could find no prejudice to P&G for me to attend.

Obviously unhappy that a court had interfered with their plan to keep plaintiffs' lawyers as separated from each other as possible, P&G then had its attorneys in Denver obtain an *ex parte* order from federal judge Sherman Finesilver, that barred the taking of the depositions in the Lampshire case if I were present. An *ex parte* order is when one side obtains an order from the court without the other side being present. Kidneigh and Kaufman were not present because, as P&G knew, they were in New York meeting with Tierno preparatory to going to Cincinnati to take the depositions.

After learning of Finesilver's decision, I located Kidneigh and Kaufman's whereabouts through their secretary. They were meeting with Tierno at Cormack's Roadhouse near Tierno's home in Bergen County, New Jersey. Kaufman told me later that when the bartender came to their table to tell Kidneigh he had a phone call, Tierno became excited. "Nobody knows I'm here," he said. Suspecting that P&G operatives had somehow tracked him down, he asked the Denver lawyers: "How did they find out?"

Tierno was much relieved when he learned I was calling and how I located him. According to Kaufman, Tierno, in the fashion of someone fearing possible attack in a public place, had picked a table in a corner without windows, and he had then sat in the chair with his back to the wall.

Kaufman also reported that Tierno was obviously a brilliant microbiologist and, most importantly, one whose beliefs could not be compromised. "He comes off somewhat eccentric and a little excitable, but he knows what he is talking about." He told me that our contacting Tierno had spurred the latter to begin active research into exactly why Rely caused *Staph aureus* to produce the deadly toxin.

But the question remained: How would Tierno hold up in court? Would it be his brilliance or his eccentricity that made the biggest impression on the jury? P&G would have the bluest chip kind of witnesses—people who are well-known leaders in their respective fields and who wrote the leading books and treatises on the subject. An example was Feinstein, the Yale epidemiologist, whom the *Encyclopaedia Britannica* would select to write about epidemiological studies in a science and health update. How good would Mike Kehm's case be in court with one unknown and excitable microbiologist from a hospital nobody in Iowa had heard of being pitted against the best scientific talent that the giant P&G could put together? The contest seemed far from equal. But there were other areas of imbalance. Mike Kehm's sole financial resources came from his job as a service manager at McGrath Pontiac, and P&G's profits in ten minutes exceeded Mike's income for the whole year. My support staff consisted of two young lawyers just out of law school plus one legal assistant who, until recently, had been a legal secretary. Arrayed against our small firm were P&G's many in-house attorneys as well as its regular outside counsel, the sixty-plus member Cincinnati law firm of Dinsmore & Shohl, together with their army of legal assistants, many of whom would come to Cedar Rapids to keep track of the thousands of court documents and exhibits.

Weighing the David and Goliath aspect of the contest between Mike Kehm and Procter & Gamble, I'd be reassured by Tierno's frequent reminders that: "There is only one truth." And the truth in this case, Tierno asserted, is that Rely tampons can kill women. I believed it, too, but would a jury?

7

"There is no question that the ecological dynamics of menstrually associated Toxic Shock Syndrome are complex, no question about that. . . . But there is, in my opinion, one bottom line and that one bottom line is the insertion of the tampon."

Philip Tierno, in direct testimony at his deposition.

I gave P&G's attorneys notice of my intention to take Tierno's deposition in New York City on August 7, 1981. Kidneigh and Kaufman asked to attend the deposition, and since it was my own witness rather than P&G employees, P&G couldn't prevent the Denver lawyers' participation.

At the last moment, though, P&G tried to cancel the deposition, claiming chaos in air travel caused by the full-scale firing of air traffic controllers by the president. Fortunately, Magistrate Hodges overruled P&G's motion.

A lot of things were going through my mind prior to Tierno's deposition. Since CDC doctors are not allowed to testify in civil cases—the government contends they have more important things to do, like fighting diseases, than appearing in court—Tierno was the only TSS scientist we knew with no ties to the tampon companies. Without an expert to give a scientific explanation for the tampon connection, even though it be only a theory, the judge might direct a verdict in P&G's favor and not even submit the case to the jury.

In his late thirties, Tierno was a relatively young man in apparent good health. I would not have been so anxious to get his deposition if I had not had an "indispensible witness" die suddenly as I was preparing for another trial. I had taken over a five-year-old case and a Mr. Burianek's testimony was vital to our side. I had a premonition to take Burianek's deposition without delay. During that deposition, the opposing attorney had asked if I intended to call Burianek at trial. I said of course, unless Burianek was in China then or "fate is unkind to him." As Burianek left the office he joked, "Riley doesn't think I'll live until the trial." That evening Burianek collapsed of a heart attack and was dead on arrival at a local hospital. That unsettling experience was the same reason I had taken nurse Sterenchuk's deposition—the only person who could prove Pat was using a tampon when she died.

There was another reason I had decided to take Tierno's deposition. I knew that juries were influenced by a person's speech and by his looks. In the same case that involved Mr. Burianek, a client of mine was hurt when a Porsche overturned on a series of twisting curves. The issue was whether the steering mechanism failed or the driver was going too fast. In this instance, the driver was a glamorous blond woman, someone the jury could easily visualize as reckless. Rather than have the driver, who had moved to Arizona, come back to Iowa to testify, I took her deposition and had a secretary read her answers to the jury. The secretary, who was prim and proper, looked like the Methodist minister's daughter, which she just happened to be. This helped create a mental picture of the driver that did not distract from the real issues.

Trials sometimes allow only a superficial impression to be gained of a witness. Kidneigh and Kaufman's description of

Tierno as a brilliant but excitable and emotional type made me worry about the superficial impression that he might have on a jury. I decided it would be better to use Tierno's deposition in court rather than have him testify in person. In addition to preserving his valuable testimony, the deposition would allow the brilliant passages of Tierno's answers to be read by someone whose appearance and delivery would not distract from the testimony—someone who would be as "establishment" appearing as I knew P&G's experts would be.

Accompanied by Kidneigh and Kaufman, I met Tierno on August 6 at the same New Jersey roadhouse where he had met weeks earlier with the Denver lawyers. Once again, Tierno sat at a corner table with his back to the wall. The microbiologist repeated his concern that he would feel safer after his deposition had been completed.

Over lunch, Tierno opened a Rely tampon and removed some small white CMC (or carboxymethylcellulose) chips which he then put in a thimble-sized glass vial. After adding a few drops of water, the synthetic chips immediately began to soften and swell out, eventually changing form entirely and becoming gelatinous and almost indistinct.

The substance felt slimy to the touch. "That's the toxin factory," Tierno said. He pointed out that the bacteria would find the substance "a favorable physical and chemical environment for toxin to produce a walling-off effect, protecting the system from phagocytic cells, which engulf or destroy bacteria if they have access to them."

Kaufman questioned how the toxin could get out of the walled-off area if the white blood cells could not get in. "The difference in molecular size is the answer," Tierno explained. The scientist pointed out that there are several factors involved besides the walling off and the fact that the CMC chips are food. "The pH rises during menstruation, which means a less acid environment is more favorable to development of bacteria. A tampon is a foreign body in a vagina." He read what the Elek experiment showed about foreign bodies and infections. He then handed us a copy from a textbook on infectious disease which stated that one hundred *Staph aureus* cells impregnated on a single suture implanted in human skin caused more infection than five million cells of *Staph aureus* injected into the skin without a foreign body being present. "That's the foreign body effect," he said.

I asked Tierno why tampons, which had been foreign bodies since their invention in the 1930s, hadn't caused TSS until the last few years. Tierno explained that a combination of factors was responsible, including the damming up of the menstrual blood and debris, which tampons didn't do originally. But, most importantly, Tierno contended, was that the older tampons did not contain the new synthetic materials, such as polyester foam and CMC, which created a new and different environment ideal for toxin production.

The next morning, we picked Tierno up at his home and headed south for the city. My direct examination went well. Tierno was relatively calm and articulate in his explanation of the world of microorganisms. He explained how his interest in TSS had been piqued by his wife's question as to why she had not gotten TSS despite her use of superabsorbent tampons. He related how he took a Rely tampon apart and was amazed to find how the tiny CMC chips reacted first with water and later with blood and plasma. He told about the October 10, 1980, open letter to P&G in order to help them find answers to the TSS mystery. He had hoped they would do the necessary research to confirm the hypothesis that he had arrived at in his rather simple experimentation.

He had pointed out in the letter that the coagulation that occurred when sterile water was added to the chips was even greater with the addition of human plasma or blood. He noticed that the longer the incubation period, the greater the effect of coagulation. He had told P&G that the polyester component formed a complex within itself by trapping nutrients, consisting of blood, tissue, cellular debris and so forth, in its matrix, thus allowing the staph enzymes to coagulate that complex, especially on the outside, and in effect walling itself off from its environment. He had suggested to P&G that this would protect the *Staph aureus* from phagocytic cells, or cells that engulf and consume foreign material, as well as from the ecological competition of other resident and transient microflora. He likened the blood-soaked Rely tampon to an agar medium used in laboratories to culture bacteria. In effect, he said that Rely tampons acted as a culture medium dish, or petri dish, and that the tampon became a complex of hundreds of "toxin factories" or "toxin chambers." He had proposed eliminating CMC, polyester and similar substances from superabsorbent tampons and expressed the hope that his preliminary research would be further explored.

He described how P&G had sent a representative, by the name of Widder, out to see him and had suggested that he apply for a P&G grant. However, Tierno's mother had just seriously injured herself and needed to be cared for by the Tiernos, and in addition, Tierno was getting ready to change his job from director of microbiology at the Goldwater Memorial Hospital and move to a new position in clinical microbiology at University Hospital, also part of NYU Medical Center. He testified he did nothing more by way of experimentation or research until we contacted him two months earlier, when he had resumed his experimentation and found that the CMC chips could be eaten by certain bacteria that were known to be present in the vaginal flora of some women. He testified that this was original research on his part with respect to the CMC in Rely tampons but that it was known in the literature that CMC would be a substrate, or food, for bacteria as early as the 1950s. He gave the opinion, as an expert, that Rely tampons play a role in the development of menstrually associated Toxic Shock Syndrome:

> "There is no question that the ecological dynamics of menstrually associated Toxic Shock Syndrome are complex, no question about that. There is no doubt that there are many parameters, many factors that are involved. But there is, in my opinion, one bottom line and that one bottom line is the insertion of the tampon."

Tierno concluded his direct testimony by stating that his experiments were simple and that they should have been done by P&G before putting Rely on the market.

> "Knowing the microflora of the human vagina, both before, during and after menstruation, I believe these microorganisms should have been tested against any product that is put into such an orifice, especially as it relates to possible substrate or food stuff value."

It was noon when I had concluded my direct examination of Tierno and the deposition was recessed for lunch. Tierno was interested in how he had done. I was able to say truthfully he had been excellent. We all cautioned him against letting this praise go to his head since Woodside would certainly try to get his goat in the hope that Tierno would say something intemperate.

Tierno did not have to wait long to be baited by Woodside. Deliberately confusing Tierno's hypothesis about "toxin factories" with Tierno's actual tests showing how bacteria broke down the CMC chips into liquid form, Woodside referred to the latter as a theory. When Tierno told him he wanted to be very clear as to what Woodside was talking about when he used the word *theory*, Woodside replied that he was talking about the liquification of the CMC chips. Tierno snapped back:

> "That is not a theory, sir. . . . That is a fact."

When Woodside tried to make the point that liquification could occur in the laboratory (*in vitro* testing) but that Tierno would have to test further to see if it would occur in the human vagina (*in vivo* testing), Tierno disagreed with him:

> "Not necessarily. If I take a gun and shoot a glass and take a gun and shoot you, I have a reasonable ability to know that I am going to put a hole in you as I am in the glass. If I use that as an analogy."
> "That may be true with a gun—"
> "I just use that as an analogy."

Kidneigh, Kaufman and I agreed that the deposition had gone reasonably well. Tierno had not followed our suggestion to remain calm and ignore Woodside's effort to ridicule him. But he had not let Woodside dissuade him from his opinion that Rely tampons increased the risk of TSS, and I knew that would get us to a jury.

Back in Cedar Rapids, I called Schlievert, the UCLA researcher and protégé of Galask, hoping that the microbiologist had developed an explanation of the tampon mechanism or, at least, would put his seal of approval on Tierno's work. The interview with Schlievert, who had left UCLA and was then at the University of Minnesota, was anything but encouraging. While admitting that he had not read Tierno's report, Schlievert ridiculed him and his contention that the breakdown of CMC would be a factor in toxin production. He told me that he didn't think CMC broke down. He quickly added that if it did, it broke down into glucose, which was known to inhibit toxin production by *Staph aureus*. He told me that Tierno sounded like a crackpot.

I told Schlievert I'd like to see him debate this crackpot.

Schlievert laughed. "In a debate with me, Tierno would lose going away."

Our conversation jolted me.

I had no trouble accepting a certain lack of objectivity in members of my profession or the parties to a legal contest. But, somehow, I'd always held the notion that scientists lived in another world—a world in which scientists, unselfishly (and relentlessly), sought the truth and let the chips fall where they may.

When I pointed out that Tierno held a responsible position as an assistant professor and chief clinical microbiologist with New York University's Medical Center, Schlievert answered that he had not been able to find Tierno listed as a member of the American Society of Microbiologists (which I later learned he was) and that he hadn't heard of Tierno until the last few days.

I brought up CDC I and II and Osterholm's Tri-State Study, hoping Schlievert would at least endorse them. Schlievert replied that he didn't know whether he accepted the studies or not:

> "Let's say you go to a ball game and they serve hot dogs there. And all of a sudden, the next day you, your kids, and your wife and a hundred and fifty other people there get hepatitis. Okay, and they trace it back to the hot dogs so they go to one of the big hot dog companies and shut their plant down. And then, two days later, they discover it was the relish they were using, and it didn't have anything to do with the hot dogs at all. Now that kind of thing happens all of the time."

I could not help but ask if Schlievert had a grant from P&G. He admitted that he did, that he had grants from the National Institutes of Health and the Minnesota Medical Foundation as well. What was more, he was expecting one from Kimberly-Clark, the manufacturers of Kotex tampons. I hung up the phone and added another name to the one-sided lineup of experts that P&G and the other tampon companies could pit against Tierno.

PART
THREE

Corporate
Conduct

8

"Don't initiate discussion of Toxic Shock Syndrome"

P&G's directive to their
sales representatives who
called on doctors.

When it appeared that the Kehm case would be one of the first TSS cases to come to trial, P&G decided to commit as much time and effort as it would take to win it in hopes that their victory would psychologically intimidate other TSS victims, causing them to fall in line and settle their cases cheaply. Ignoring the research grants, the company eventually spent more than a million dollars directly defending the Kehm case. A quarter of a million dollars was spent just for secret mock trial rehearsals that P&G would hold in Lincoln, Nebraska, two months before the Kehm trial began.

A few weeks before taking Tierno's deposition in New York, I deposed a number of P&G executives and other personnel who were involved in the development of Rely tampons. The highest ranking official was Charles Fullgraf, group vice president of P&G. The other P&G witnesses were those deposed by Kidneigh and Kaufman in Cincinnati earlier in the summer of 1981, when P&G had obtained the order from the Denver judge Finesilver banning my participation.

I learned little from the depositions of the P&G officials
except that the company wasn't admitting anything. One
P&G loyalist, Gordon Hassing, who had a Ph.D. in biochemistry, even refused to concede that *Staph aureus* was associated
with TSS. While those scientists who were beneficiaries of
P&G's grants would still question whether tampons were involved, by the time Hassing gave his deposition no reputable
scientist had any lingering doubt that *Staph aureus* was the bacterial culprit. Hassing's self-righteousness irritated me.

I did gain concessions that P&G gave no warning about
tampons and TSS between the time in June when the company learned about the tampon association and Pat Kehm's
death on September 6, 1980, but I already knew that. P&G's
Fullgraf, a moon-faced man in his late sixties, who looked like
everybody's notion of a kindly grandfather, made several admissions. He acknowledged that it would have cost no more
than a penny or two per package to put special warning labels
on the Rely boxes that had already been printed. He admitted
that P&G's sales force in the field had experience in applying
special labels to P&G products while they were on the grocer's
shelf. He said such occasions involved cutting prices on the
product to meet competition, and he agreed that such a practice could have been implemented by P&G's in-field sales representatives if the company had decided to mount such a warning
campaign. Fullgraf also conceded that P&G knew about the
Imboden TSS suit filed in California in early August and that
P&G officials in Cincinnati reviewed video tapes of newscasts
about that suit and other reports of TSS with Rely tampons.

I pressed the P&G officials on why no warning was sounded
for all American women since the company's own studies
showed that the rest of the country lagged far behind California in awareness of TSS. Their answers were all the same.
P&G had no scientific evidence of an actual connection and
did not have it even at the time of the depositions. The CDC
and other epidemiological studies were only circumstantial evidence and subject to flaws in design and execution.

I considered the depositions successful if for no other reason than that I was forewarned that P&G was playing hardball and I could not expect any help from company personnel in proving even the simplest scientific proposition connected with TSS.

"Better to know it now and be ready to meet the burden of proof alone," I told Michele. "They're not even conceding Pat Kehm might have died of TSS."

I took some satisfaction that the P&G executives were forced to come to Iowa to give their deposition. P&G's action of going to Judge Finesilver in Denver to keep me from sitting in on the Kidneigh and Kaufman depositions in Cincinnati resulted in an order from federal court that this deposition would be held in Cedar Rapids and not in Ohio.

The decision whether to require a protective order was up to Magistrate Hodges, to whom the United States District Court judge, Edward J. McManus, routinely assigned all responsibility for discovery problems. McManus, who is a former lieutenant governor of Iowa and was appointed to the federal bench in 1961 by President Kennedy, lacked prior judicial experience. Most observers felt the appointment was a consolation for McManus's unsuccessful effort to win the governorship of Iowa on the same ticket with Kennedy in 1960. Prior to becoming a federal judge, he had divided his career between part-time politician and county seat lawyer. As a federal judge, he soon inaugurated some pretrial procedures that were eventually recognized as farsighted, but that aroused some bitterness among older lawyers who were set in their ways and who found the new rules time consuming.

The two common complaints about McManus were that he wasn't learned enough in the law to sit as a federal judge and that he wasn't accessible to lawyers when they wished to argue a motion or discuss some other matter either before or during a trial. With respect to the competency criticism, McManus was being judged against his predecessor, Henry

Graven. Graven's decisions were well-written, scholarly tomes, and he was recognized throughout the country as one of the outstanding federal district judges. McManus relied heavily on bright law clerks and people like Hodges to advise him. And, while McManus had not distinguished himself as a legal scholar, he had avoided any embarrassing judicial blunders. On the bench, his impatience with the pace of a trial would often find him peering over his reading glasses to ask the lawyers curtly to move along. This was the judge who would try the Kehm case.

I recognized some advantages to being in federal court, however. One was that the Eighth Circuit Court of Appeals, whose decisions McManus would have to follow, had adopted a minority position among the circuit courts on a rule of evidence that would let the Rely recall come into evidence. In state court, evidence of the recall was not then admissible. Though the recall would not be conclusive proof that the product was defective, it would be evidence that the jury could consider on that issue. A second advantage was that McManus's impatience with long trials would tend to keep P&G from bringing an army of scientists to the stand to prove the same point. And, after all, it was P&G, not Mike Kehm, who had the money to array such an army.

When I refused to submit to a protective order, it became Hodges's task to rule whether one was needed. As I saw the situation, Hodges had three choices. He could assume P&G's claim regarding trade secrets was wrong (a mere smokescreen) without looking at the documents, he could examine each document and rule on it, or he could give P&G its way and avoid both the possibility that there were some confidential or trade secret documents and the time that it would take him to find out.

He took the latter course, and on August 14, 1981, McManus signed an order granting P&G's application for a protective order. Under the terms of the protective order, my staff and I would be in contempt of court if we showed any document that P&G had marked confidential to anyone outside the firm, including other TSS victims or their attorneys. We could show the documents to an expert witness we employed (such as Tierno), but only after first notifying P&G and giving P&G the right to object if the expert had ties to a competitor. Any expert that P&G didn't successfully challenge would have to sign the nondisclosure agreement so that he couldn't share the information with other scientists in his field—an oppressive inhibition that might slow scientific research into the causes of TSS. The revision about experts being disclosed for P&G's approval or objection gave P&G an extra advantage. It would learn the identity of all the experts that the plaintiff's attorney had talked to whether he decided to call them as witnesses or not.

Having no choice, I signed the protective order. I then asked my daughter Sara, who had returned to college but was now home for the summer, to join Michele and a recently hired secretary on a trip to Cincinnati to carry out the document inspection. On Sunday, August 17, 1981, the three young women drove the five hundred miles from Cedar Rapids to Cincinnati where, the following day, they presented themselves at the reception desk of Dinsmore & Shohl, on the twenty-first floor of the Fountain Square Plaza in downtown Cincinnati. A short time later, they found themselves in a large building nearby, where they were free to begin their search for needles in a haystack of 600,000 pieces of paper.

The three women had gone to Cincinnati with instructions to check out complaints of illnesses resembling TSS, documents relating to development, testing, and marketing of Rely and activities of P&G during the summer of 1980. When they asked to see documents relating to those areas of inquiry, they were told that P&G would not provide them with specific documents. Instead, boxes of documents would be brought to them one at a time. For three days, they waded through box after box of generally insignificant documents dealing with such things as the manufacturing schedules for Rely at the various P&G plants or tests on rats. On the fourth day of their search, Sara overheard a P&G employee refer to an index.

When Sara asked to see the index, the P&G employee said she would check with her superiors. After doing so, she told Sara and Michele that the index was "attorney's work product" and they would not be permitted to see it. Furious, Michele called me long-distance. When I found that three days had been wasted and that P&G wouldn't produce requested materials covering a special subject, I, too, was outraged. I told Michele I would call off the search of documents and ask the federal court to intervene. I immediately contacted the local P&G attorney and told him:

"Those turkeys in Cincinnati have had their way in refusing to produce documents here in Cedar Rapids, and we've been forced to go to Cincinnati to see them, and when, at no inconsiderable expense, I send three people out there for a week, P&G won't produce the documents—they just tell our people they're free to look for them in a warehouse of papers. This makes a mockery of discovery, and if you can't shape them up out there, we're going to let Hodges hear about it."

The phone call worked, and while P&G wouldn't let my staff people see the index, its employees did produce boxes containing the complaint files and other specific subjects that we requested. Several hundred documents that we hoped would help prove P&G officials turned their backs on their customers once they learned of the tampon association were copied and brought back to Cedar Rapids.

In reviewing the documents, I was chagrined to discover that Dr. Jeffrey Davis, Wisconsin's public health officer, had become the recipient of a substantial grant from P&G and, even before that, had, I felt, put personal gain ahead of the public interest in delaying public release of a report that had been bought and paid for by the taxpayers of his state. Entitled "TSS Study by the Wisconsin State Health Department," the report was authored by Davis and other public employees. Davis had sent a draft copy to the CDC for its comment and review. The CDC, in turn, had provided the FDA with a copy of the study, and it was then placed in an FDA administrative file. When Davis learned that the manuscript might be available to the public under the Freedom of Information Act, he protested and demanded its return. The HEW, in a November 13, 1980, memo to the FDA, noted that Davis "would not have submitted this study to CDC had he known the study would be publicly disclosed." Davis told the FDA that he would be happy to provide them with a copy of the study when it was published. The desire to wait until publication rather than reveal findings important to the fight of disease at an earlier time seemed immoral, if not illegal, where a private investigator was concerned. When the investigator, however, is a public health officer on the public payroll, as Davis was, it appeared to me to be a breach of fiduciary duty which, if not deserving of criminal punishment, was grounds for censure at least.

I noted that in a further effort to get Davis to release the data for inclusion on the FDA docket on a proposed rule for warning labels on tampon boxes, HEW again "discussed with Dr. Davis his position concerning public disclosure of the Wisconsin study. His position had not changed." Accordingly, HEW asked that the Wisconsin study not be returned to the FDA administrative file. Davis again told the FDA that he would provide them with a copy of the study when it was published.

In other documents obtained in the P&G search, I noted that Dr. Michael Osterholm, Davis's counterpart as state epidemiologist in Minnesota, took the same position regarding FDA use of the publicly funded Tri-State Study (an Iowa, Minnesota and Wisconsin TSS study paid for by the state health departments of the respective states).

In a February 9, 1981, letter to the acting commisioner of the FDA, Osterholm acknowledged that "it is in the interest of public health to make our study results part of the public record as soon as possible so that interested persons may have access to them." However, Osterholm, pointing out that he and his staff were in the process of preparing a final manuscript on a TSS study, demanded the preliminary draft he supplied FDA be returned since he did not want the public to have access to it. Osterholm was too subtle to state in a letter to the FDA why he did not want it to be published. However, an FDA memo of April 3, 1981, regarding a telephone conversation with Osterholm lays it out:

> "Dr. Osterholm called to follow up my conversation with the Commissioner of Public Health of Minnesota about new data concerning Toxic Shock Syndrome. I had asked the Commissioner to discuss with Dr. Osterholm, who has conducted a study on tampons and their relationship to TSS, the possibility of making results available to FDA for public release in connection with FDA rulemaking on a TSS warning label.
>
> Dr. Osterholm had earlier expressed a concern that release of the data in connection with the rulemaking could adversely affect chances of having the study published. He has, however, contacted two journals and has been assured by at least one of them that release to FDA and the public in connection with the rulemaking will not be considered 'publication' and will not adversely affect that journal's review of his study.
>
> Having reached that understanding, Dr. Osterholm said that he had no objection to use by FDA of his data and will make them available to us. I said that the Associate Commissioner for Regulatory Affairs would be in touch with him to discuss the form in which the data would be received and released."

I noted that complaints to P&G averaged ten to fifteen a month. Many involved Rely tampons coming apart and parts sticking to the vaginal wall. Some involved complaints of infection and vaginitis with a rash. Several interested me because they sounded like people who had TSS.

One in particular stood out. It involved a twenty-five-year-old housewife and mother of two children who worked as a long-distance telephone operator for Northwestern Bell and whose husband was employed by a small printing firm. Long before science had begun to look at the tampon and TSS connection, this young Omaha housewife had figured out that Rely tampons could kill her.

Sue Myers had been pregnant with her first child in 1979 when the free sample box of four Rely tampons arrived in the mail. On Wednesday, September 5, 1979, six weeks after her child was born, Myers began her first menstrual period. Since she still had the free sample of Rely tampons, Myers thought that she might as well try them. She liked them enough to buy a box at the grocery store. She had never used Rely tampons prior to this and had never had any problems with her periods. About midmorning on Friday, September 7, 1979, two days later, she began to feel "sluggish and just kind of rotten but nothing I could put my fingers on yet." By evening, she started vomiting and having diarrhea. She remembers having to throw up in the sink because she was sitting on the toilet and having diarrhea at the same time. This continued throughout the night, and she thought she had the flu and made no connection between her illness and the Rely tampons that she continued to use. She took her temperature, and it was about 103 degrees. She was eventually hospitalized on Saturday, September 8, 1979, in the intensive care ward with a blood pressure at one time as low as 48 over 38 and a pulse of 140. On the seventh day of her hospitalization, whole areas of skin around the tips of her fingers, hands and toes peeled off. Her doctors were puzzled by her illness and finally guessed she had some strange type of viral infection. The Rely tampon that she had been wearing on admission to the hospital had been removed and discarded because of a general policy against tampon use during hospitalization—a policy that probably saved Sue Myers's life.

After her release from the hospital on September 15, 1979, Myers's strength gradually improved, she went back to work at the telephone company and life returned to normal in her household.

She began to experience the same symptoms the second day into her next period. As she sat in the bathroom vomiting and with diarrhea, she thought to herself that this was the same exact thing she had had before, and she was near tears because her illness the month before had been so horrible that she was terrified at the prospect of repeating it. As she gathered her senses, she kept trying to think "what on earth have these two occurrences in common. There has to be something. I just can't be getting sick for no reason at all."

Myers says that it was then that it "just hit me. I was using a different tampon than I had ever used. The only time I had ever used them was both the times that I got sick. I had just started using Rely tampons that last period, and I started using them again this time, and I started getting sick exactly a day and a half each time exactly—I mean almost to the hour."

Myers then removed the Rely and started using a pad. Her illness continued but she didn't get as sick as the first time, probably due to her realization of what was causing her illness and the decision she made to stop using tampons.

On October 11, 1979, Myers called P&G because she assumed that her illness had been a result of an allergy to some substance used in Rely, and she wanted to identify this substance or chemical so she could avoid it if it appeared in other products. Sue recounted her illnesses during September and October's menstrual periods and pointed out that the use of Rely was the only common factor. In an undated P&G interoffice memo written by a Doris Kuzzler, Kuzzler noted that Myers was "quite pleasant and responsible and seemed very intelligent." Kuzzler also reported that the Nebraska woman was "especially interested in learning the composition of Rely, and I gave her this information."

The information Kuzzler gave Myers was misleading at best. Kuzzler implied that the product was made of rayon and cotton—which was not true. Kuzzler's memo didn't state

what she told Myers the ingredients of Rely were, but a
P & G letter written to Judith Labowitz of Munster, Indiana,
offers a clue as to what was probably said. Labowitz's teen-
age daughter, Rebecca, had contracted TSS in April 1980,
and her mother had written to P & G on August 4, 1980,
inquiring, among other things, about the components of Rely.
On August 28, 1980, P & G wrote Labowitz and stated that
"the super-absorbent fibers in Rely are made from natural
cellulose. Cellulose has been used in tampons and other forms
(rayon and cotton) for many years."

The statement was deceptive. The superabsorbent fibers
in Rely were chemically treated synthetics known as carboxymethylcellulose, CMC for short. CMC was no more a
natural cellulose than is plastic or cellophane. Moreover, the
references to cotton and rayon implied that Rely was made
of these two well-known and harmless substances but "in
other forms." The deception didn't work with Myers, however. She was convinced that Rely tampons were made of
something other than cotton and rayon since those materials
were no strangers in her life and they had never caused her
an allergy in all of her contacts with them.

I phoned Sue Myers, who was willing to speak freely to me
about her illness. I told Myers about Pat Kehm's illness, her
use of Rely tampons for the first time and her death four days
later. We spoke of the similarities in their cases, their age, their
having two small children and their use of Rely for the first
time after safely using other tampon products. Myers said she
realized that she had had TSS after she read a description of
the illness in a newspaper story in 1980. She then spoke to her
treating physician who agreed that was what she had had. The
physician eventually wrote a case study about his patient in
the *Journal of the Nebraska Medical Society*.

In the fall of 1981, I traveled to Omaha and met with
Myers at her home. She was a pleasant, pert and vivacious
young woman. I noticed that she had a tendency to talk
rapidly (something I assumed she might have acquired in

her job as a long-distance telephone operator), and thinking of Tierno, I wondered if all of my witnesses would give the impression to the jury of rapid-fire excitability.

But there was no mistaking Sue Myers's sincerity, which was topped off by the fact that she was foregoing a claim against P&G for her TSS illness even though she had a valid one. "I got well, so I'm not going after them," she said. Myers mentioned that she still had the Rely box and showed it to me. She agreed to keep it until the Kehm trial was over and promised to come to Cedar Rapids and tell the jury what had happened to her in the fall of 1979.

Unquestionably, the most incriminating documents were those showing that from the time P&G learned of the tampon association late in June 1980, until Rely was recalled from the market three months later, P&G issued specific instructions to its sales force not to bring up the subject of TSS when they called on doctors. I thought about my interview with the emergency room physician who had examined Pat Kehm on September 5, 1980, the night before she died. Pat had been so ill she vomited more than once in the emergency room. The physician had admitted that his diagnosis of flu was wrong because he had not heard of TSS at that time and he didn't recognize her symptoms. If the emergency room physician had heard of TSS and treated Pat Kehm for it that night, she probably would have lived. Instead, a critical twelve hours or more passed while the Rely tampon remained inside her and the deadly toxins continued to be produced and to attack her organs and tissue.

P&G knew that TSS wasn't well known even among the medical community in the summer of 1980, and they not only took no steps to educate doctors through their sales force but they issued specific orders to keep the lid on. I wondered, what kind of corporate mentality are we dealing with?

9

"The exchange of information about TSS has dried up. It's a result of the P&G grants. . . ."

Dr. Bruce Dan, former CDC epidemiologist, February 8, 1982.

December 8, 1981, was a good day for TSS victims and their lawyers. December 9 wasn't. On the eighth, the *Wall Street Journal* carried a front page story that appeared to put an end to P&G's claim that there was no scientific evidence linking Rely tampons to TSS. Dean Rotbart of the *Journal's* Cleveland bureau wrote that laboratory tests showed substantial toxin production by *Staph aureus* in the presence of all tampons but not in the presence of cotton, wool or other controls. The story reported that Rely tampons caused the highest amount of toxin production of all tampons. Rotbart quoted Merlin Bergdoll, a University of Wisconsin expert on *Staphylococcus aureus* toxin, as saying:

> "My preliminary indications are enough for tampon makers to be concerned about."

It was just like Phil Tierno said: "There is only one truth." Thank God, I thought, the truth is out at last.

Bergdoll's findings would make the case a lot simpler. It would still be necessary to convince the jury that Pat had had

TSS, but scientific evidence that the new tampons, especially Rely, act on the bacteria in a way that causes toxin production when cotton and wool don't, should make it easier to prove that Rely tampons are defective and that it was the tampon and not the IUD that caused the toxic shock infection. It would explain why the original cotton tampon invented by Dr. Haas didn't cause TSS.

Unfortunately, the next day, the *New York Times* carried a story in which Bergdoll refuted the *Wall Street Journal*'s story. He denied the remarks attributed to him that his findings were significant. Instead, he claimed that the results were not only preliminary but inconclusive. The *Times*'s story quoted P&G as reporting that Bergdoll's toxin did not produce TSS symptoms in laboratory animals. Pat Schlievert was quoted as suggesting the problem might be with individual traits in the woman rather than the tampon. It appeared that Bergdoll's studies would be of questionable value to TSS victims because their author was now renouncing them as meaningless.

Nonetheless, I tried to obtain the Bergdoll data. However, Magistrate Hodges accepted P&G's claim that the results were preliminary and were privileged as a research product that could not be released without consent of the researcher. Hodges ruled that P&G wouldn't have to produce any information it received from the scientists it funded unless the scientist was submitting the information for publication in a scientific journal. But he did order that P&G would have to furnish to me the results of any in-house research that was supplied to P&G's expert witnesses who would testify in the Kehm case. P&G ignored this last order.

What I would not find out until much later was that the Bergdoll research was far from preliminary. P&G had duplicated the results in their own labs. Moreover, on March 25, 1982, just eleven days before the Kehm case would come to trial, Bergdoll sent updated findings to P&G that confirmed the work he had done in the fall of 1981 (the subject of the *Wall Street Journal* article).

When I finally saw the Bergdoll data—nearly two years after the Kehm trial—I found that Rely tampons caused enhanced toxin production twenty to one hundred-fold over other tampons. Cotton and wool, as the *Wall Street Journal* story had reported, did not cause toxin production, nor did a control that Bergdoll used. The jury would never have the benefit of this highly damaging evidence.

P&G's witnesses would swear under oath that they knew of no scientific evidence suggesting a connection between Rely tampons and TSS. Yet they knew that far from the federal courthouse in Cedar Rapids, the Bergdoll data were safely filed away in Cincinnati, and they also knew they didn't have to worry about my cross-examining them about it.

On January 15, 1982, P&G filed its list of expert witnesses. In the Kehm case, as in other TSS cases, P&G waited until as close to trial as the particular court would permit—in order to allow the plaintiff less opportunity to conduct an investigation into the witnesses's backgrounds and to prepare and take their depositions. The experts cited by P&G included Herbert L. Ley, Jr., M.D., a former FDA commissioner, who would testify that Rely testing exceeded FDA requirements for drugs; Alvan Feinstein, M.D., the Yale expert on epidemiology, who would testify that the CDC and other studies were flawed and could not be relied upon; Dr. Tommy Evans, of Wayne State University, who would testify that Rely was safe; Peter Reilly, professor of Chemical Engineering at Iowa State University, who would testify that Tierno was wrong about CMC being broken down by bacterial enzymes; Dr. James Todd, the discoverer of TSS, who would testify about the origin, recognition and treatment of TSS; and Dr. Charles Helms, of the University of Iowa College of Medicine, who was a coauthor of the Tri-State Study and would testify about the epidemiological studies. P&G also listed a number of in-house experts who would testify tampons did not cause TSS and that Pat Kehm did not have TSS. But I noticed that Pat Schlievert, for some reason, wasn't listed as a P&G witness.

Even without Schlievert, it was clear that Tierno and I had our work cut out for us. Fortunately, within days after assessing the unequal battle of plaintiff's and defendant's experts, help would arrive. I discovered that Bruce Dan had left the CDC and might be available to testify as to his knowledge of the disease and the two studies called CDC I and CDC II.

I wasted no time phoning long distance to ask Dan in Atlanta to review Pat Kehm's medical and hospital records since P&G was claiming both that Pat didn't have TSS and if she did die of it, it was the IUD and not the tampon that was responsible. I also wanted the former CDC expert to testify on TSS matters in general. Dan agreed to review Pat's records for his standard fee of $300.

A few days later, Dan called to confirm that Pat Kehm had TSS. "There are a few things not documented such as the rash, but that often is missed by the examiner, and if her husband saw it, I don't doubt it for a minute because everything else falls into place perfectly."

I told Dan I was relieved to hear that. P&G's Dr. Elizabeth McKinivan, an in-house medical doctor, said Pat's records proved otherwise. Since the CDC's briefing of P&G officials in June of 1980, Dan had met most of the people concerned with Rely including McKinivan. He told me he wouldn't expect McKinivan to say anything less, she was a "company man."

I suggested that it would be helpful to meet with Dan, so on February 7th, my wife and I flew to Atlanta. The next morning Dan called from the lobby of our hotel. I invited him up to our room to meet, and Dan said that was a good idea because the tropical birds in the lobby were driving him nuts with their squawking. A few minutes later, a slender, dark-haired, young man was at my door. My immediate impression of Dan was a college activist type, undoubtedly a result of his droopy mustache and blue jeans. I automatically size up a witness to decide what kind of an impression he might make on the jury. I noticed that from the side, Dan reminded me of the debonair old movie star, Zachary Scott. He didn't look like your typical establishment M.D., let alone someone who had held such high responsibility for the public health.

I asked Dan to tell me about himself, his work at the CDC and his prior background and training.

Dan talked about TSS, its discovery and its association with menstruating women in 1980. I was particularly interested in how the toxin damaged the woman's body and caused death. Dan believed the toxin damaged the walls of cells, causing the contents to spill out. "Red blood cells, which carry oxygen to the other cells of the body, are damaged, and with the oxygen transport system affected, you see the labored breathing, the shock lung, the frothing and congestion in the lung caused as the capillaries are breaking down." Dan's explanation as to why so few women got TSS was the same as Tierno's—"the woman must have *Staphylococcus aureus* in the vagina, and only 5 to 15 percent of the women do, which cuts the potential down. Then," he continued, "it must be a particular strain of *Staph aureus* and this cuts it down a lot further. Lastly, the woman must not have been previously exposed to the toxin so that she hasn't yet developed antibodies and that means that we're talking about a relatively small class of women."

I asked Dan why women would get repeat bouts of TSS in succeeding menstrual periods, and Dan theorized that the toxin apparently overpowered the immune system of the woman, something that a Professor Fred Quinby at Cornell Medical College would demonstrate in tests on baboons in the following year.

Dan was friendly, articulate and self-assured. He told me about the tense moments at the FDA meeting in September 1980, when the FDA threatened a recall of Rely if P&G didn't take voluntary action to withdraw the product. He told how P&G's chief counsel, Powell McHenry, objected to the word "recall" being used, and the FDA's young attorney, Nancy Buc, said she didn't care what they called it as long as the tampon was off the market. "She facetiously said they could call the recall a banana for all that she cared. It was really bizarre after that. All these important government people and

P&G big shots sitting around the conference table and using the word 'banana' in place of 'recall' as the high level debate about Rely's future continued," Dan chuckled.

Dan also talked about the dramatic moment when P&G failed in its attempt to prevent public release of CDC II: "Tom Laco [the executive vice president of P&G] was practically down on his knees while his eyes moistened as he looked at me and said: 'You realize what this means to P&G? What if you're wrong?' I looked him right in the eye and replied: 'Mr. Laco, what if you're wrong? What if it would be your own daughter?'"

I told Dan about an FDA memo I had seen that was written by a Lillian Yin, who seemed to be friendly to P&G's side in the summer of 1980. Dan laughed: "Yin is incompetent. The FDA put her over in tampons thinking nothing ever happens with tampons. It was the worst place for her to be in when TSS broke out." Dan said she was very jealous of her turf and when CDC I showed that tampons weren't as safe as everybody thought, Lillian couldn't or wouldn't believe the study. Dan asked if I had seen the FDA bulletin that was sent to all doctors in July. I told him that one of the doctors who treated Pat Kehm on the day she died—the only one who had heard of TSS—said that he had gotten the bulletin. The doctor had saved it and later shown it to me.

"Well," Dan continued, "the FDA fought us on issuing a statement, and we had to write the bulletin for them ourselves and pull strings to get it sent out. It was the only public pronouncement by the FDA on TSS in the summer of 1980."

"It's bad enough that P&G and the other tampon manufacturers let greed or fear keep them quiet that summer, but it's outrageous that our own government worries more about the welfare of the tampon companies than American women," I told Dan. "If things had been different, Pat Kehm would be alive today."

Dan then related a story about FDA commissioner Jere Goyan and Yin. At a meeting of the CDC and FDA during the summer of 1980, discussions centered on how government officials could obtain critical information on the components of the various tampons. After some time had passed with various officials speculating on how to acquire the much needed information, Yin spoke up: "I have that information in my files." When Goyan asked to see it, Yin replied: "I can't release it, it's confidential FDA information." At this point, an exasperated Goyan brought the house down by exploding: "For God sake, Lillian, I am the FDA. You can show it to me!" Dan recalled that Yin then relented and provided her boss and the CDC officials with the data they had been seeking for months.

I told Dan I had not been impressed with Goyan. Goyan spoke to the Tampon Manufacturers Association and applauded P&G for what he called P&G's selfless act of withdrawing Rely. "I've seen the official minutes of the two FDA and P&G meetings that led to the recall," I told Dan, "and it was about as voluntary as KP duty in the army."

"Well, you have to remember that the commissioner of the FDA is appointed by the president and that it's a political plum," Dan replied. "If the FDA commissioner doesn't make enemies for himself and the FDA, it reflects well on his boss in the White House. Besides, we'd accomplished what we wanted. Rely was off the market, and it made everybody feel good to give P&G a pat on the back."

"I've seen some letters from yourself, Shands and other CDC doctors that also suggest that P&G acted responsibly in removing Rely. P&G's attorneys will pounce on those statements at trial."

"That was all cosmetic," Dan replied.

"Speaking of Shands, what kind of a person is she?"

"Kathy is tremendous. She's smart and honest. You've got to understand that all of us were under a lot of pressure during the summer of 1980. We had an epidemic on our hands. Women were dying, and we had to find out why. We were working from 7 a.m. to 3 a.m., seven days a week, researching, answering calls from doctors in the field who were treating TSS cases, answering questions from the news media, appearing on network news programs and so on. Kathy handled her job beautifully and showed tremendous grace under pressure." Dan added: "One of the tampon companies offered me a lucrative job when I left the CDC. I turned it down—it sounded too much like they were trying to buy me off."

"I got a little irritated with Shands not long after I got this case," I told Dan. I described an interview that Shands gave about TSS after the recall of Rely, in which she seemed to be playing down the tampon connection. She told the audience that women were at a greater risk of getting injured in a car accident en route to the drug store to buy a tampon than of getting TSS from tampons.

"While that may be statistically true in this age, in most places you have to drive a car as a practical matter, but you don't have to use tampons. One is a virtual necessity and the other is a convenience. Remarks like hers tend to lull women into a false sense of security. Instead, she ought to be crusading to make women more aware of the consequences of TSS rather than pacifying them."

Dan said that Shands was only trying to put things in perspective. "The incidence of TSS is low, and for most women it's not a threat. Kathy was probably trying to reassure women that they could continue to use tampons, especially since Rely was off the market, but I'm sure that she would want everyone to know that there is a risk."

The conversation returned to the technical side of TSS. I asked Dan if he agreed that TSS might be host specific, meaning that in the case of TSS, only humans might get it—just as dogs don't get the human disease of mumps and humans don't get distemper. The reason I was curious about Dan's opinion was that P&G's witnesses were emphasizing the fact of Koch's Postulates (a scientific test) not being fulfilled with respect to TSS and that, until that was done, there was no scientific certainty that the toxin suspected in TSS cases was actually the causing agent. As I understood Koch's Postulates, a scientist must extract the toxin from the patient and produce the same symptoms when the toxin is injected into a laboratory animal and then extract the toxin from the same animal.

Dan agreed that it might be that only humans can get TSS so that tests of laboratory animals with TSS toxin would not bring about TSS symptoms.

"Well," I said, "if laboratory animals are immune, then we will never be able to scientifically establish a toxin that is responsible for TSS since we can't test toxin in humans. It will just be theoretical or based on circumstantial evidence like the CDC studies."

Dan acknowledged that might be the case and then revealed that he had volunteered to inject the toxin into his own arm to prove that it caused the symptoms of TSS.

"Weren't you afraid of the consequences?" I asked.

"You bet I was, but I proposed diluting it to an infinitesimal fraction, where only a mild reaction would occur at worst."

I asked what happened.

"Dr. Foege, who is the CDC director and assistant surgeon general, wouldn't give permission. He said he'd be drummed out of medicine if he approved such an experiment."

The talk turned to other aspects of the tampon connection. I asked why bacteria produces toxins. Dan said one reason was to drive off other microorganisms competing for territory and food. He explained that it was defensive in that instance. I relayed what Tierno had said, that one single cell of bacteria, given a limitless amount of food, could multiply to the point where its weight would equal that of the planet earth in twenty-four hours and of a thousand such planets in merely two days.

Dan told me of a CDC test in which *Staph aureus* survived on dry Rely tampons for up to six weeks while they were dead in a week or two on other tampons. The latter was the maximum length of time *Staph aureus* should live on a dry surface without nutrient sources available.

By then, it was only a formality, asking Dan if he'd testify in court that Rely tampons caused Pat Kehm's illness and death. Dan said exactly what I wanted to hear, that he would testify. I told him that up until now, the contest had been a little one-sided, with only Mike Kehm and one relatively obscure microbiologist against P&G and all of the big names in TSS research.

I told Dan I had seen a number of P&G documents referring to him in less than complimentary terms. I described one
document that said Dan dominated a CDC discussion with
P&G officials and wouldn't let some technical subordinates
speak up, and in another, a P&G official sarcastically commented that Dan was on a crusade so that he could one day
look back proudly and tell his grandchildren how he had put
Rely off the market and saved all those women's lives.

"You didn't play ball with them like other people did—in
and out of government," I asserted. There was another P&G
memo that outlined a strategy to deal with the TSS crisis by
cultivating and influencing the CDC with respect to its TSS
investigation. "Even after they struck out with you and Rely
was off the market, they were still trying to seduce you and
Shands." I showed Dan a P&G memo that was dated October
17, 1980, from Geoffrey Place to P&G vice presidents Butler
and Laco. In it, Place discussed P&G's "fundamental strategy" of weaning Shands and Dan away from the "tampon-
Rely crusade." Place stated further:

> "I would plan to achieve this by having Shands/Dan rec-
> ognize that P&G is already producing data and is com-
> mitted to further research that is important to them, their
> crusades, and their careers. Unlike their university peers,
> we are not interested in using this data to compete with
> them for scientific glory and career advancement. In fact,
> given an appropriate climate of interaction between CDC
> and P&G, access to our data will enhance their ability to
> be seen as leaders of the crusade against TSS."

"Well, it doesn't show a very high regard for our motives,
does it?" Dan said.

"Those university peers are the very people P&G is funding
in their claimed effort to advance science," I replied. "They
don't show much respect for their university researchers either, do they?" Before Dan could respond to the rhetorical
question, I asked him what he thought about P&G's funding.
Dan told me that, as a scientist, he was saddened to see what

was taking place in TSS research since P&G had starting lavishing money on TSS researchers.

"In science, we have, ordinarily, a free exchange of information. If one researcher has a question in his research, he can pick up the phone and find out directly what the other researcher knows and what he is doing. It's an attitude of mutual respect and trust," Dan continued. "But the exchange of information about TSS dried up. It's a result of the P&G grants and the realization that P&G doesn't want anything about TSS out until the company clears it first. It's a shocking commentary on the integrity of science."

"The scientists claim that they aren't being bought off," I countered, "because none of them are getting P&G money directly in salaries. The grants could only be used for laboratory equipment, personnel staffing and that sort of thing—salaries for their people working below them."

"That's baloney," Dan replied, "The currency of scientific research is not money, it is laboratory equipment and staffing. That's where the prestige is, that's what the scientist wants. The salary increases from the institutions that employ the scientist will follow if he gets the research grants and, especially, if the new laboratory equipment and so forth lead to publication of research findings. But, even if the salary increases wouldn't automatically happen, the scientist still wants the laboratory equipment and staffing. It's well known. Ask their scientists. Ask Jim Widder, who is in charge of P&G grants, whether he agrees with the proposition that the currency in research is not money but laboratory equipment and staffing." I wrote the question down verbatim.

Heading toward Lenox Square, where we were to meet Nan for lunch, I brought up the subject of Wayne Williams. Williams was in jail in Atlanta awaiting trial for the murder of eighteen to twenty black boys. Williams continued to express his innocence, but the killings had apparently stopped since he had been placed behind bars. I said the dramatic falloff in TSS cases after Rely was withdrawn was equally persuasive circumstantial evidence of the Rely connection. Yet, I speculated that if Williams were innocent, the real killer could be holding off on further murders to make the case look good against Williams so they wouldn't be out looking for him.

"No," Dan disagreed, "a person capable of the cold-blooded murders of those children is so irrational and obsessed that he is both incapable of refraining from further violence and incapable of doing something rational like you suggest."

"P&G claims that the drop-off in TSS cases after Rely was taken off the market is a result of doctors losing interest in reporting the disease," I told Dan. "May I assume that is as farfetched as the theory that the real murderer has stopped killing in order to finger Williams?"

"You may," Dan replied.

10

"I pray that you and that large corporations take your responsibilities to heart and warn the general public of what has become a serious and, in my wife's case, fatal illness due to lack of knowledge."

Mike Kehm, in letter to Dr. James Todd,
P&G grant recipient, March 27, 1982.

The trial of the Kehm case was scheduled to begin in federal court in Cedar Rapids on April 5, 1982. While Mike Kehm and I were anxiously looking forward to getting the case to trial, a legal maneuver by another plaintiff's lawyer threatened to postpone the trial indefinitely. He had filed a petition to consolidate all Rely TSS cases under a federal procedure known as multidistrict litigation, or MDL. If the petition were granted, all cases in federal court would be assigned to one judge who would supervise discovery conducted by a committee of lawyers representing TSS victims. MDL is used frequently in federal court in multidistrict cases such as plane crashes. It is being used in the claims against Union Carbide in the Bhopal, India, disaster. The purpose is to eliminate repetitious depositions, as well as to avoid duplicative demands on many different judges to settle identical points of disagreement on discovery and other pretrial issues. All cases would be held in abeyance while the discovery and pretrial work were carried out.

I had no idea of the complexity of TSS litigation nor the expense involved when I took the case. Consolidating depositions and similar discovery activities and then spreading the cost over all victims would make the cost to each TSS victim minimal—something that P & G would not like to see happen.

As much as I agreed with the wisdom of using MDL jurisdiction in Rely TSS cases, I was opposed to it in the Kehm case for two reasons. One, it would come too late to help defray our expenses as discovery was virtually completed, and two, it would postpone our trial date for possibly two years.

I decided to appear in Washington, D.C., at the hearing set for oral arguments on whether to grant the petition for MDL. I planned to ask the panel of judges to exempt the Kehm case from MDL should the judges grant the petition for MDL. Nonetheless, I was determined to tell the judges that MDL should be granted for TSS cases that were not already prepared for trial.

At the Court of Claims building, there were around a hundred attorneys waiting to argue their particular MDL cases. One of the cases involved the crash of an Air Florida airliner into the 14th Street Bridge in Washington that had occurred only a few weeks earlier. Unlike the TSS litigation, which found plaintiff's attorneys seeking MDL and the defendant P & G opposing it, here both sides wanted MDL. Their disagreement centered on whether the case should be referred to the federal district court in Washington, D.C., where the airliner crashed into the bridge, or the federal district court in Virginia, where the airliner took off for its short-lived flight of a half of a mile. The reason for the disagreement was clear to everyone in the courtroom. Plaintiffs favored the District of Columbia as the forum because it was considered to have more liberal judges while Air Florida attorneys preferred Virginia for the opposite reason.

The Rely TSS litigation was the last item on the court docket that day, and the courtroom was cleared of most of the attorneys by late morning. From the time I had left the elevator, I worried that I wouldn't get the opportunity to address the three-member court because of the large number of lawyers seeking to be heard. Before leaving Iowa for Washington, I had learned from a clerk for the MDL court that I would have five minutes to argue my position. I had timed and tailored my remarks to fit within the five minute allocation. When I arrived, a different clerk told me I had only three minutes. But, before I had time to cut my prepared remarks any further, the same clerk reappeared to announce that my time allocation had been cut to two minutes. "Two thousand miles for two lousy minutes," I thought as I began jettisoning additional points from my prepared arguments.

When my name was finally called, and with occasional glances at my wristwatch, I requested the panel to exclude the Kehm case from MDL because the case was ready for trial. However, I told the court I supported the petition for MDL because it would spare others the ordeal of discovery that my client had experienced as a result of footdragging by P&G with respect to discovery. I argued that P&G opposed MDL because it wanted to keep plaintiffs in the dark and separated from the activities of other TSS plaintiffs. I then told the court how P&G had prevented my attendance at the depositions of P&G officials that Kidneigh and Kaufman had set up in Cincinnati. I explained that P&G's real purpose in getting the order from Finesilver in Denver was to carry out its strategy to keep plaintiff's lawyers apart. MDL in TSS cases, I said, would frustrate that strategy. On the 120th second of my allotted time, I sat down.

Most lawyers, including those representing P&G, felt the panel would grant the MDL petition. The consensus was wrong. While the Lampshire case was in progress in Denver and a month before the Kehm case was to come to trial in Cedar Rapids, the panel handed down its decision. There would be no MDL for any TSS cases. P&G had won another battle—it could continue to keep the "enemy" divided and in the dark.

It would be a costly defeat for TSS victims, many of whom would have to spend considerable sums of money duplicating the investigations and research that had already been done by myself and Kidneigh and Kaufman. But the panel's decision would turn out to be more costly for the taxpayers as well, since the Rely TSS litigation would occupy the time of judges and juries in many different federal courts. By contrast, the Air Florida litigation was concluded "with unusual speed" according to the Washington Post News Service. Four years later, the Rely TSS litigation drags on.

In February, I was in Colorado for our firm's second annual ski trip. That was also the time I set aside to take Dr. Todd's deposition. When I reached Children's Hospital, I was directed to a conference room where P&G's attorneys and the court reporter were waiting. As soon as I arrived, word was sent to Todd, and he appeared moments later.

I had seen a P&G memo, dated August 27, 1980, in which Todd had been quoted as telling a P&G investigator that tampons did play a cofactor role by creating a functional abscess in the vagina. I wasted no time getting to the heart of the matter. I asked Todd if he still believed that tampons played a cofactor role in the cause of TSS in menstruating women. Yes was Todd's answer. Did Todd recommend immediate removal of the tampon upon the appearance of any of the clinical signs of TSS, such as nausea, diarrhea or fever during menstruation? Yes, again, came the reply. Had there been a drop-off in TSS cases since the withdrawal of Rely from the market? No, said Todd, not in Colorado.

Then I asked Todd about his grants from P&G. When had he made formal application for a P&G grant? October 1980 was his answer. When did he write the editorial in *Pediatrics* that was favorable to Rely and in which he had referred to the controversy as "toxic schlock"? The month following, Todd admitted. How much money did the grant pay him? The first year was $240,000, Todd replied, and the second year was $163,000, for a total of $403,000. But, Todd volunteered that none of it went to him personally. It all went to the Children's Hospital of Denver, he said. Thinking of Dan's comment about the currency of research, I asked if any of it went for laboratory equipment, staffing and salaries for his assistants. Yes, came the answer—all of it. Was Todd asked to find out why tampons were associated with TSS? No, came the answer.

What was he to do to earn the grant? To conduct active surveillance of new TSS cases in Colorado so that none would be overlooked, Todd replied. It was as I had assumed. P & G knew that active surveillance would reveal more TSS cases in Colorado than were identified when Rely was on the market. P & G could then exploit the fact that TSS cases had not dropped in number since Rely was taken off the market.

I quizzed Todd about his being called a P & G man by scientists who had heard about his large P & G grants and his expression of support for the P & G position. I could tell by Todd's reaction that he was sensitive about his P & G ties. In the *Pediatrics* editorial, Todd had said that CDC I caused physicians and the public to be inundated with media coverage of what might be called the "toxic schlock syndrome." He claimed that CDC II confused the public because it indicated TSS might be linked to a specific brand of tampons:

> "The public was stirred to such hysterical levels that Toxic Shock Syndrome became a household word and Rely tampons the culprit."

"Do you mean," I asked Todd, "that it did more harm than good to tell women about tampons and TSS in 1980 than if they had been continued to be left in the dark?" Well, no, Todd conceded. He admitted that there was a great deal of misinformation, but it was possible that some lives were saved and some illnesses avoided as a result of both the information and misinformation about tampons and TSS in 1980.

It was at this moment that I changed my tactics. I wanted Todd to say that he had told anyone who asked him early in the summer of 1980 that tampon use should be discontinued immediately upon early signs of TSS. At that time, Todd was probably the only nationally recognized TSS expert. If Todd had made such statements, then I would argue to the jury that P&G would have learned of this if they had only taken the trouble to contact this nationally recognized expert on TSS in June when the CDC had warned of the tampon association with TSS. If P&G had checked with Todd, they had no excuse for not warning their women customers to remove the tampon upon the first TSS signs.

I could argue to the jury that if Pat Kehm had been so warned by P&G, she would be alive today. I planned to tell the jury the warning could have been placed on the box or put on television and in the newspapers. P&G could have sent warnings through the mail—the same way they mailed the free samples of tampons. But, I had to persuade this witness who had financial ties to P&G to say what I wanted him to say—and not what P&G wanted to hear.

When I asked him what he told the press in the summer of 1980, Todd had answered that he told them that toxic shock occurred in males as well as females and that tampons didn't cause TSS, *Staph aureus* did. P&G was happy with Todd's answer at that point. So I suggested to Todd that women hearing the TSS expert's views in the summer of 1980 would be relieved by a statement that tampons didn't cause TSS. Realizing that I was backing him into a position where he would be morally responsible for tampon-related injuries and deaths in the summer of 1980, Todd said that that wasn't his intent. Pressing the guilt trip aspect for Todd if he answered wrong, I asked him:

> "There will be evidence in the trial of this case that my client's wife had two small children, one born three months

before she died of Toxic Shock Syndrome after using
Rely tampons for the first time beginning on September
2, 1980. What did you say or publish that would have
given her or her physician any warning of this association,
Doctor?"

Todd answered:

> "What I told the press was that if there is an association
> with tampons that I personally felt that the association
> was not confined to Rely tampons, and that if I was going
> to advise people, it would be, "if you have a fever and are
> using a tampon, you should remove it and seek medical
> attention."
>
> "You were saying that, then, in the summer of 1980?"
> I asked.
>
> "I was saying that in the summer of 1980. Once, as I
> pointed out, that June article came out," Todd acknowl-
> edged.

As the deposition ended I concluded that, overall, Todd's
evidence would not help P&G that much. Todd would emphasize that TSS was seen in nonmenstruating women; his
first study, the one that was published in *Lancet* in November
of 1978, included boys who had the disease and, certainly,
tampons couldn't be blamed for their sickness. He would also
testify that TSS was still a syndrome and not a disease because
the cause of TSS had not been scientifically proven, that even
the toxin suspected of causing the symptoms may not be the
correct one and that while tampons have been associated with
TSS, that "association" isn't "causation" and that it has not
been scientifically established that tampons cause TSS. But,
two important admissions had been obtained.

The first was that while Todd couldn't prove it, he held the
opinion that tampons played a role in the development of TSS
in menstruating women and, second, that as early as June 1980
he had told anyone who asked him that tampon use should be
discontinued immediately upon the sign of fever.

The importance of the first admission was obvious. Despite P&G's attack on the epidemiological studies and the lack of scientific proof of a tampon relationship, the best known expert on TSS and P&G's most heavily funded researcher held the view that tampons played some kind of role in TSS. The second point was equally important because of the time of Pat Kehm's death. Had Pat been told to remove the tampon and seek medical help when the flulike symptoms appeared two days before her death, she would probably be alive. P&G hadn't contacted the nation's only authority on TSS in June of 1980 after notification by the CDC about the tampon association. They didn't contact him in July either but, instead, mailed 2 million free samples of Rely to American households. They waited until the end of August 1980 to contact Todd and learn his views on tampons and TSS. I now had my strong argument: had P&G shown concern for its consumers, it would have contacted Todd in June, learned of his recommendations to remove the tampon upon the early symptoms of TSS, warned Rely users and Pat would not have died.

Not counting travel expenses, the deposition had cost Mike Kehm about $1,300, $1,000 of which were Todd's charges, at the rate of $250 per hour, to answer my questions and to read the transcript of the deposition. While I regretted the mounting expense, I felt Todd's admissions well worth what the doctor charged.

When my client (Mike Kehm earned $11.50 per hour as the service manager at the Pontiac agency) sent Todd his personal check for $1,000 on March 27, 1982, he wrote a letter with it, pointing out that his children would have had the opportunity to grow up knowing their own natural mother's strong love and devotion if P&G had put a warning on the Rely package:

> "Instead, they can visit her grave because P&G didn't think the situation was important to warn her or others. . . ."

He expressed the hope that if Todd would find himself in a situation in the future where people are becoming seriously ill and are dying that he wouldn't joke about media coverage of the disease. He closed:

> "I pray that you and that large corporations take your responsibilities to heart and warn the general public of what has become a serious and, in my wife's case, fatal illness due to lack of knowledge."

Todd was disturbed enough by Mike's letter that he would write a lengthy letter in response. Mike received it after Todd had testified in the Kehm case as a P&G witness. The letter began by expressing understanding about his bitterness but soon revealed an annoyance about my client's comments:

> "It may be comforting to villify me and imagine me to be callous and biased, but I am afraid I do not fit into such a convenient niche."

Todd claimed that he would be testifying in the Kehm case "reluctantly so the jury will have the most accurate information available to allow them to make a very difficult decision," but Mike Kehm knew all about Todd's reluctance.

After the Todd deposition had ended, I headed for the law offices of P&G's Denver counsel for the deposition of James Widder, the P&G microbiologist in charge of TSS research and the man responsible for awarding the P&G research grants. Widder had dispensed money to scientists all over the United States, even as far away as Hawaii, in the case of Dr. Helen Mellish, and, internationally, as far as Denmark, in the case of Dr. Gorm Wagner. He had made several unsuccessful trips to New York City to see if he could interest Tierno in taking P&G money and, as it would turn out, would try to persuade Tierno to do so as late as the eve of the Kehm trial.

Widder was short and very stocky. He wore his hair in a crewcut and peered through horn-rimmed glasses. His expression was serious but not unfriendly. He appeared nervous about the prospect of giving his deposition. There was a delay in Widder's deposition because the court reporter wasn't feeling well. While we waited for the new court reporter, Widder and

I, in the presence of the P&G attorneys, made small talk. During our conversation, I sized Widder up as a basically honest man who would not deliberately lie or, as P&G's Hassing had done, look foolish by taking an untenable or ridiculous scientific position solely to please his employer. I suspected that Widder, like most witnesses who are partisan to a cause, could be persuaded by P&G's attorneys to put the best light on his testimony from P&G's standpoint. Sensing that Widder's nervousness would combine with his basic honesty to give unshaded answers in the early part of the deposition (before his nervousness wore off and the P&G attorneys could call him aside), I decided to go for the bottom-line answers right off the bat. I knew Widder wouldn't place more blame on Rely tampons than others. But I didn't care about that. All I wanted from P&G's top in-house TSS expert was an admission that tampons were involved or had a role in TSS despite the lack of hard scientific evidence. I began by asking a question that recognized Widder's extensive background and expertise in TSS.

> "Doctor, you have been in charge of directing the inquiry into TSS for P&G since the fall of 1980, and you have done a great deal of study and testing in consulting with others, and you've seen a great amount of research data on TSS and spent more than a year in this investigation, isn't all of that true?"

Widder answered yes. Then I followed up by appealing to Widder's sense of integrity in the pursuit of scientific truth by specifically beginning his next question with reference to Widder's status as a scientist:

> "Doctor, based on what you know and as a scientist don't you think it's probable that tampons, and I'm not picking only on Rely, but that tampons do in all probability play a role in menstrually associated TSS cases?"

To my great relief (and before P&G's attorneys could think of an objection at that point to educate Widder to hedge his answer), Widder responded:

"I think the answer is yes."

Later, I got Widder to admit that he had thought what Tierno had to say in his open letter to P&G of October 10, 1980, was "logical." At the trial, Widder would deny that he had said Tierno's theory was logical, which gave me the opportunity to impeach him by reading his deposition.

I also used the question Bruce Dan had suggested, and Widder agreed that the currency of research was not salary but equipment and staff personnel. Now, I could argue that P&G knew the way to curry favor with scientists was by offering them grants for laboratory equipment and personnel staffing and that it wasn't necessary to pay the scientist extra compensation—in fact, without direct salary compensation, the scientist would be able to convince himself that he still had his integrity, despite his interest in doing nothing to offend P&G and jeopardize his grant renewals.

After the deposition was completed, I thanked Widder and told him that he was an honorable man. I had not felt that way about the other P&G scientists, particularly Hassing. The unsought praise in the presence of the P&G attorneys did little to lighten Widder's apparent anxieties about the way the deposition had gone from P&G's standpoint. With a nervous attempt to interject humor, Widder responded, "I think I'm in trouble."

11

"P&G is systematically and scientifically supporting the search for the truth—nothing more and nothing less."

Claim in P&G press kit.

Back in Cedar Rapids, questions had to be outlined for my own witnesses and cross-examination prepared for P&G's. The exhibit list had to be assembled and decisions made as to which should be used and which were significant enough to be blown up. Legal briefs had to be drafted and the many depositions of P&G witnesses synopsized so I could contradict them if, during the trial, the P&G witnesses strayed from their earlier sworn testimony.

P&G filed a motion asking the court to keep me from telling the jury about the CDC and the state epidemiological studies. They contended the studies were hearsay and were not reliable due to various alleged biases. P&G also asked the court to admit the evidence of P&G's withdrawal of Rely as "background" only. I wasn't sure what P&G meant by "background" but I understood the second part of that request— that the judge tell the jury that the withdrawal of Rely could not be considered evidence of negligence on P&G's part or evidence that the tampon was defective. I filed a resistance to P&G's motion and awaited the court ruling.

Local federal court rules required the lawyers to exchange copies of exhibits in advance of the pretrial conference so that objections could be taken up before the trial began. At the eleventh hour, P&G's attorneys had submitted some ten thousand to us that pertained to various tests of Rely and its components. P&G hoped that the jury would be convinced—just by looking at the two dozen jumbo-sized, black three-ring notebooks—that they had engaged in extensive good faith testing of Rely. Sitting side by side for the length of a long conference table in the federal courtroom, they would be silent witnesses to the length that P&G had gone to make a safe product. With all of the seemingly more important final trial preparation to do, I didn't take the time to carefully examine the thousands of test documents in detail before the copies had to be returned to P&G attorneys. P&G had expected that.

In reviewing the test documents after the trial while the case was on appeal, I was amazed to find that many of the documents had nothing directly to do with Rely testing.

On February 26, 1982, the final pretrial conference was held, and Magistrate Hodges inquired whether the parties' clients could agree to a compromise settlement. P&G's principal attorney in the Kehm case, Tom Calder, of Dinsmore & Shohl, said that P&G would pay $150,000 in settlement of the lawsuit. Calder explained that past Iowa jury verdicts in deaths of house-wives had exceeded that sum on only one occasion. A condition of the settlement, he said, was that P&G would insist the settlement amount be kept secret. I told Hodges my client felt the offer was inadequate. Hodges asked what facts could be agreed upon to save court time proving facts not really in controversy. About all we would agree on was that Patricia Kehm died on September 6, 1980, was married to Michael Kehm, left her two daughters surviving and that P&G manufactured and sold the tampon known as Rely.

The point that Calder had raised about the compensation value in the case of the death of an unemployed housewife was a genuine concern. I explained to my client that verdicts in Iowa, a generally conservative state, were lower than usual in death cases. The jurors attitudes seemed to be that there wasn't anything that could be done to help the dead person and they weren't going to make the heirs rich. It was part of Iowa's rejection of the "world owes me a living" philosophy. I pointed out that juries will award damages for an actual economic loss—that there are many farmers on Iowa juries and that they know the value of property, such as land, and of work. If someone gets hurt or killed by someone else's fault, a jury will award whatever is necessary to make up for the income loss. But where a housewife is concerned, there is no income loss for the defendant to reimburse and juries aren't too generous about the intangibles, such as loss of love and affection. Some jurors seem to look at that kind of claim as "blood money," and in the case of young people, they figure the spouse will remarry sooner or later and that life will go on.

I told Mike Kehm that based on the past track record of Iowa juries, P&G's offer wasn't out of line for settlement purposes. Mike replied that he wasn't interested in letting P&G off the hook: "They let my wife die, and I want them to be found liable by a court of law."

The Kehm case would be the third Toxic Shock Syndrome case in America to come to trial. The first was won by Johnson & Johnson in South Carolina. The next case to come to trial was the one Kidneigh and Kaufman had filed on behalf of their client, Deletha Lampshire, who sued P&G as a result of an illness in late May 1980—a few days before the CDC began its study that would be known as CDC I. Ms. Lampshire told jurors that she suffered memory loss and depression as a result of her illness, adding, "I felt dirty, and I still do—no man would want to marry me."

The cooperation between the Denver attorneys, Kidneigh and Kaufman, and myself, had been mutually advantageous in getting our cases ready for trial. Many of the witnesses called by both sides in the Lampshire case would also testify in the Kehm case. P&G attorneys would hold back from using some of their experts in the Lampshire case, apparently thinking they had it won. They wanted to save some surprises for the

Iowa case, which they took more seriously because of the death of Mrs. Kehm. The Lampshire case was like a dress rehearsal for P&G's attorneys. They would be able to try out tactics and strategies that could be either used or discarded for the Kehm case.

It was imperative for someone to monitor the Lampshire case to cut into P&G's advantage in trying a TSS case before I did. I didn't know and wouldn't find out until a year and a half later that P&G was not limiting its trial preparational advantage to the Lampshire case. P&G paid a California firm $200,000 to stage three mock trials of the Kehm case in Lincoln, Nebraska, giving P&G attorneys and witnesses a chance to rehearse and be critiqued over and over by professional coaches and psychologists. Lincoln was selected because its population came closest to matching in socio-economic demographics the type of people who lived in northeast Iowa, the area from which the Kehm jury panel would be selected. The P&G attorneys would obviously benefit from the professional coaching and critiquing by the California firm and the comments of the three sets of Lincoln area laymen who were picked to hear the evidence in the three mock trials.

After each of the three mock trials, the jurors would be carefully debriefed to find out which witnesses they liked and disliked and why, which evidence they felt hurtful to P&G, which evidence they felt helpful and what style or approach they approved or disapproved of. After each mock trial, the P&G witnesses and attorneys would attempt to modify their performance in line with the critiquing by the jurors and the professional coaches. Each jury would vote on how they felt the case should be decided.

Whether the modification during the mock trials may have gone so far as to constitute perjury will probably never be revealed. However, there is now evidence that lends credence to the conclusion that P&G set out in the mock trials to sell its testimony just like it sells soap—with carefully tailored scripts that are structured from research in the marketplace as to what captures the attention of the public and what does not. Moviegoers who thought that James Mason's fictional portrayal of a lawyer for a powerful defendant in *The Verdict* was unrealistic and exaggerated might reconsider in light of the conduct of P&G and its defense of the Kehm case.

Another method employed by P&G in the defense of the Kehm case would not come to light until publication in the summer of 1983 of an issue of *Trial Diplomacy Journal*. Psychologist Thomas Sannito wrote in the magazine how he and his wife, a human behavioral scientist, were employed by P&G to help pick the jury and then to monitor the jurors frequently during the two and one half week Kehm trial. Sannito explained that P&G attorneys "made use of the information provided to alter strategy with witnesses and to enhance the effects of the final argument." Is it possible to "alter strategy with witnesses," based upon juror reaction to earlier testimony, other than by having the later witnesses change their testimony to conform to what the experts think influenced the jury? Sannito may have meant that the line of questioning of later witnesses focused on those issues that seemed to interest or impress the jurors and to ignore those that didn't, but he didn't elaborate in the article.

Because I could not spend the time necessary to attend the entire Lampshire trial, Michele and my wife, Nan, monitored parts of it. The travel expense involved in the monitoring was one more financial burden that Mike Kehm would have to bear, but the opportunity to observe the witnesses for both sides would help offset to some extent the advantage that P&G's attorneys and witnesses gained from actual participation in the Lampshire case, not to mention the three secret mock trials about which I was unaware.

P&G fought the Lampshire claim on two major grounds. It argued that Ms. Lampshire did not have TSS and, if she did, that Rely did not cause it. The jury spent nearly twenty hours in deliberation before reaching an incongruous verdict— Rely was defective but Ms. Lampshire was entitled to no damages. P&G's public relations department quickly issued a news release congratulating the company for not having been found responsible for Ms. Lampshire's illness but regretting the jury verdict about Rely. The news release insisted that Rely was not defective.

I always felt the Lampshire case should not have been the first to go to trial against P&G—principally because of the fear that Ms. Lampshire's largely subjective claims would not go over well with the typical jury. I recognized that jurors have trouble accepting either bizarre or subjective complaints from plaintiffs, and Ms. Lampshire had both. To make matters worse for her claim of permanent injury, Ms. Lampshire appeared outwardly to be in excellent health, and she was frequently being interviewed by the media. Her ingratiating smile appeared often in the newspapers and on television, and despite the judge's instruction to avoid news coverage of the trial, it would have been virtually impossible for the jurors to miss those pictures at one time or another. Another complicating fact for Ms. Lampshire's claim that she had suffered long-term effects was her election as student-body president at her high school the year after her illness.

The jury verdict answered "No" when attorney Tom Calder, alluding to her high school election, asked: "Does that sound to you like a woman who has been held back?" Ironically, a study of a group of TSS victims published after the Lampshire verdict lent credence to Ms. Lampshire's complaints. Dr. Karen A. Rosene and a team of other doctors reported in *Annals of Internal Medicine* in June 1982 their findings of persistent headaches, memory lapses, difficulty concentrating and dizziness in post-TSS cases.

In any event, lawyers who had tried unsuccessfully to persuade Kidneigh and Kaufman to delay their case until a pattern of victories for TSS victims could be established against P&G, breathed a collective sigh of relief that the Lampshire verdict was no worse than a standoff. *Time* magazine called the result a "verdict on tampons but the impact on toxic-shock cases is unclear." *Time* noted that: "The next major trial, involving a death case after the use of Rely, begins in two weeks in Cedar Rapids, Iowa, and the plaintiff's lawyer in that case,

Tom Riley, went to Denver to watch the Lampshire trial. If he had not known it already, he learned that toxic shock mysteries now include legal uncertainty as well." Ms. Lampshire's motion for a new trial was eventually granted by Judge Feinsilver on the basis of the apparent contradictory nature of the verdict, and the case was then settled for an undisclosed sum.

My wife and I had dinner with Bruce Dan following his testimony as an expert witness for Ms. Lampshire. Dan's performance on the witness stand was one of the most impressive I had ever seen, and I told him so. Dan had been examined by Calder's assistant Frank C. Woodside III, M.D., who had left his law practice at Dinsmore & Shohl long enough to graduate from medical college.

While relaxing over wine and raw oysters at the basement bar of a popular Larimer Square restaurant, we discussed the sensitive points that Woodside might raise in the Kehm case after he regrouped for another attack on Dan. I told the doctor that Woodside would be certain to hit him hard on the three thousand dollar fee he was charging for each day in court: "The insinuation will be that you are making a lucrative career out of testifying in TSS cases. My thinking is that I will bring what you charge out on direct examination, so as to steal their thunder."

The former CDC expert replied, "I am not afraid of talking about my fees. I'll tell them the truth." He explained to me that he charged a high sum for three reasons. First, he didn't have the time to participate in every TSS case, and by charging a high fee, he wanted to discourage people from asking him to get involved in their cases. Second, he devoted unpaid time consulting with doctors from all over the country for information about treating their TSS patients. Finally, when he was not answering telephone inquiries he was writing articles on TSS, which provided no income, and he was also writing a book on TSS. "The court fees help me live while I do these things," he concluded.

I asked Dan if he had anything else to bring out under direct examination. During a deposition in another case, Dan was asked if tampons caused TSS and he had replied, "Of course not." He said that the lawyer had failed to ask a follow-up question, "Do tampons cause TSS in menstruating women?" Dan said that if the lawyer had, he would have answered, "That's a different question, and the answer to that question is yes."

I promised to send Dan a complete list of the questions I was going to ask on direct examination. If any of the questions didn't make sense, Dan was to let me know. "I've decided to have you lead off our case because I want to start off with a strong witness," I told him. "I'll have you lay out the TSS story in its entirety and educate the jury to the world of microorganisms just as I had to educate myself to get ready for trial."

The next day Dan returned to Atlanta, and I left for Cedar Rapids, leaving my wife behind to continue monitoring the Lampshire trial.

The jury panel list for the Kehm case had arrived from the clerk of court while I was in Denver. The jurors were mostly small-town and rural people who would be even more conservative than a representative cross section of Iowa. There were some relatively large cities in the area, but these towns were hardly represented on the panel. Cedar Rapids, the largest city, with a metropolitan population of about 150,000 people, had only six jurors on the panel of forty. On the other hand, Epworth, with a population of only 1,200, had three jurors on the list. The jurors' occupations were equally conservative— many held jobs that were allied to management and, presumably, would be sympathetic to a company being sued. If the juror was a blue-collar worker, it was at a minimum wage job in a nonunion business, where the worker would not be exposed to the liberal attitudes within union-organized plants.

In actuality, jury selection is really juror rejection. In the Kehm case, McManus would have fourteen names drawn and then the lawyers for each side would reject three; the remaining eight would constitute the jury.

Because Judge McManus drastically limited the amount of time for jury selection, I decided to consult with Hale Starr, a behavioral science expert from Des Moines. Starr would assess prospective jurors by analyzing their body language, clothing, voice and mannerisms. She would be able to draw a psychological profile in a relatively short time.

There was another reason I wanted to employ Starr. In a recent Teamsters trial, I had asked if any juror had ever said or heard anything critical of the Teamsters Union. Not a single hand went up, even though all but one of the last Teamster presidents had been convicted of felonies and the then current president was under indictment. In the past, I've expressed a criticism of the Teamsters on occasion and I was certain so had all those jurors, but the way McManus limited jury selection, I was unable to discover which jurors had deep-seated prejudices that could not be overcome.

I had sent Starr the Kehm jury panel list. Starr agreed with my assessment that the luck of the draw had delivered a conservative jury panel as a whole.

As the trial date approached, I received a telephone call from the Minnesota epidemiologist, Michael Osterholm, who was the principal author of the Tri-State Study. Osterholm had been less than supportive when I had called him by telephone the summer before. So I was surprised by his offer to help. Osterholm asked why plaintiffs' lawyers were not calling on experts, like himself, but were approaching people like Tierno. I said Tierno had come off well in the Lampshire case since the jury verdict found Rely defective as Tierno claimed. It became clear that Osterholm now felt ignored in the TSS litigation after having made news a year earlier with a release of the Tri-State Study, and he wanted very much to be asked to testify in the Kehm case. "You're making a mistake if you're relying on Tierno. Schlievert has agreed to testify for P&G and he is going to tear Tierno apart. That's one of the things I'm warning you about."

Osterholm's comment didn't worry me. Schlievert had been added as a late witness to P&G's list of experts, but the court had ruled, at my request, that he could only testify as a rebuttal to Dan, who had been a late edition to the Kehm's expert witness list.

I had no intention of calling Osterholm; he was too close to Schlievert, who was definitely partisan to P&G, and I didn't intend to call an expert to the stand who felt as hostile to Tierno as Osterholm did. Even if I stuck to asking Osterholm about the Tri-State Study, which was generally helpful to our side, P&G's attorneys would get around to asking Osterholm his opinion of Tierno and Tierno's theories. It was tolerable to have P&G's experts ridicule Tierno. I could shrug my shoulders to the jury and, by body language, ask: "What do you expect?" It would be a total disaster to have one of my own experts do so.

A month before the trial was to begin, my secretary, Roberta Lyle, told me she had just heard on her car radio that the Mayo Clinic released a study showing there was "nothing wrong with Rely tampons." I immediately phoned Tierno in New York City and asked if he had heard the news about a Mayo study. Tierno had heard the report on the "Today Show" that morning and had checked it out. "It is nothing to worry about, Tom. They've got it all wrong." "Nothing to worry about?" I asked. "Out here, the Mayo Clinic is considered the closest thing to medical perfection since Christ raised Lazarus from the dead." Tierno told me to calm down. "All these guys did was test the components of each tampon, including Rely, and found each nontoxic by itself. That's not new. We've known all along that the components won't poison you, it is what they do to the staph to allow it to produce toxin that makes the tampon dangerous."

Still, I wondered aloud, how many potential jurors had been influenced by the story? The trial was now only days away. In anticipation, P&G's public relations personnel, accompanied by an executive from a local advertising firm hired by P&G for the Kehm trial, paid calls on all newspapers, and radio and television stations. A press kit was provided to the various news departments, and the P&G delegation offered to arrange interviews with P&G personnel and witnesses. The kit contained a supposed background briefing on tampons and TSS. It contained misrepresentations, such as a statement that claimed that the Utah study, in which twelve of the twelve TSS cases, or 100 percent, were tampon users compared to only 80 percent among the controls, "showed no statistical association between tampon use and Toxic Shock Syndrome." The sample wasn't large enough to have scientific validity, but P&G had altered that fact to claim that the Utah study showed tampons were innocent.

P&G's press kit applauded the company for "funding TSS research" since "P&G is systematically and scientifically supporting the search for the truth—nothing more and nothing less." My blood pressure hit 210 when a newsman told me about this claim. "The only trouble with that 'research' is that P&G doesn't intend to share the truth with anyone until they have all TSS litigation behind them," I told the newsman. I suggested to the newsman that he ask P&G for a copy of the Bergdoll research that P&G funded and that P&G refused to let anyone see.

P&G also arranged to have a number of sample P&G products dropped at Cedar Rapids residences on the eve of trial. It may have been a mere coincidence. If it was not, it was an expensive effort, since only six people from Cedar Rapids would be on the starting panel of forty prospective jurors.

As P&G approached the Kehm trial, its strategy had been fully implemented. It had frustrated the discovery rules and had suppressed scientific research about TSS. Its attorneys and witnesses had been carefully rehearsed in three mock trials in Lincoln, Nebraska, and now, on the eve of trial, they were pleased about the timing of the report from the Mayo Clinic that tampon products, including Rely, contain no toxic materials. But they were even more pleased by the verdict of the third Lincoln mock jury—the one that had heard the evidence after P&G's attorneys and witnesses had ample opportunity to polish their performances. Unlike the first two mock juries, the verdict of the third jury was for P&G and against the Kehms. P&G was now ready for trial in Cedar Rapids.

PART
FOUR

Fighting
the Giant

12

*"In view of the fact that the tampon was
thrown away and disposed of, there is no
way that we can show whether or not
that tampon had, and prove that that
tampon had, any bacteria in it, can we,
from a clinical point of view?"*

P&G attorney's question to Dr. John Jacobs
on cross-examination.

When I arrived at the federal courthouse for the beginning of
the Kehm trial, the spectators' benches in the courtroom were
crowded—and they remained generally so throughout the two
and one half week trial. People apparently felt some sense of
participation in history-in-the-making—minor history, perhaps, but history nonetheless. For here, in Cedar Rapids, one
of America's best-known corporations was accused of taking
the life of a young mother by manufacturing a defective product. The bizarre result in the Lampshire trial may have kindled
interest in the Kehm case. Perhaps, more than anything else,
it was the mere craziness that one could die from a tampon—
sort of like getting mortal wounds in a pillow fight.

When Mike Kehm was introduced to Hale Starr, she told him to remove the vest of his three-piece suit. She said vests make men look too much like bankers—the wrong image for a deserving plaintiff. P&G attorneys had won a toss of the coin flipped by the deputy clerk of court to decide who sat where. Mike, Todd, Michele and I took our places at the side of the counsel table nearest the jury. Lawyers don't like that side because their backs are to the jury as well as the witness if the table is used to write upon. The opposite side of the table was preferred because a lawyer would be facing the jury, the witness and the table all at the same time.

Four P&G attorneys sat down on their side of the counsel table, Calder and Woodside from the Dinsmore & Shohl firm and two Cedar Rapids attorneys who were hired as local counsel. A third Dinsmore & Shohl attorney sat near the counsel table with legal assistants flanking her on both sides. Additional P&G lawyers and legal assistants were present in the courtroom and more would appear from time to time. P&G's command headquarters was in an office building a block away. Cedar Rapids isn't large enough to have an office furniture rental firm, so P&G went out and bought what it needed—desks, typewriters and other office equipment—for their delegation of attorneys, legal assistants and secretaries. When Mike commented on the discrepancy between the number of attorneys on each side of the table, I told him not to worry, only one of P&G's platoon of attorneys could talk at once.

McManus asked if the parties were ready to proceed, and when both sides answered that they were, he instructed the deputy clerk to call fourteen names from the jury panel list. When those chosen had taken their seats in the jury box, McManus explained to them that the lawsuit involved a claim against P&G for the death of Patricia Kehm allegedly as a result of getting Toxic Shock Syndrome from using Rely tampons. He asked some general questions of the group, such as: Had they or their spouses ever used Rely tampons? Had they formed any opinions about the case? Then McManus turned the questioning over to me.

One of the first questions I asked was: "Have you, or any close member of your family or close friend ever been involved in an accident in which someone else was killed or injured?" Such an experience might cause the juror to identify with P&G, which stood accused of causing Pat Kehm's death. A young woman answered that several years before, a bicyclist had struck her car and was killed. I asked if a claim had been filed and she indicated that it had been settled out of court. I then asked if that experience would make it difficult to be impartial in this case since it also involved a claim for wrongful death. While the juror said that she did not think it would, I noticed a flinching as if her body were saying it would while her voice said that it would not. I started to ask the juror if she had resented being sued by the child's parents, but before the juror could answer, McManus declared that she had said she would be fair and that that was enough. I met with similar rulings when I tried to probe jurors' attitudes—attitudes that might predispose them one way or the other. Because of the brevity of the questioning, I had only a hazy idea of the type of people I was dealing with.

There was an exception—Betty Beauregard, who lived on a farm that adjoined one owned by the parents of Steven Warbasse, one of the two local P&G attorneys sitting at the counsel table. The attorney had grown up on his parents' farm and was well acquainted with the Beauregards. Questioning of Mrs. Beauregard brought out that the Beauregards and the attorney's parents still socialized. Ordinarily, I would have struck Mrs. Beauregard from the fourteen, but this seemed to be a situation of the lesser of two evils. I felt there were other jurors who would be more harmful to our side. One strike was used on a nun whose career, body language and verbal response suggested both to myself and to Starr a "turn the other cheek" stoicism that would hardly be conducive to adequate compensation—an attitude of "you get your rewards in heaven, not on earth." She also vaguely reminded me of the farmer's wife in *American Gothic*. A second strike was exercised on the schoolteacher who was sued for the bicyclist's death. The third strike eliminated a juror whose background suggested possible empathy toward manufacturing concerns.

Mrs. Beauregard worked with the local community action program, and the analysis by Starr indicated that she was honest and compassionate. Aside from her relationship with a P&G attorney these qualities made her an ideal juror from our standpoint. Warbasse was particularly surprised we kept his family's friend on the jury, but I believed her when she said she would not let that relationship interfere with doing justice. I also sensed that there might be the slightest feeling on her part that the young neighbor boy had gotten "a little too big for his britches." The P&G attorney, a former farm boy, was now given to wearing three-piece suits and driving around town in a rented Cadillac.

The eight member jury that was eventually sworn to try the Kehm case was equally divided between men and women. It consisted of an eighteen-year-old corrections officer, who would volunteer for the job of foreman, a Cedar Rapids radio assembly worker, an unemployed roofer from a rural area, the wife of a small-town bank president, an employee of the Waterloo Parks Department, Mrs. Beauregard, a self-employed upholsterer and a secretary (both from Cedar Rapids).

The first words I spoke to the jury were: "On September 2, 1980, Michael Kehm's wife, Pat, used Rely tampons for the first time. Four days later she was dead." I went on to claim that her death was unnecessary and was a result of Procter & Gamble's selling Rely tampons to American women without complete testing and failing to warn of the symptoms of Toxic Shock Syndrome after having been notified of the problem by the Centers for Disease Control two and a half months before Pat Kehm's death.

P&G's opening statement set the tone for its defense of the case. Acting on the premise that the best defense is a strong offense, P&G's attorney attacked everything from the validity of the epidemiological studies of the CDC to the diagnosis of TSS by her physicians as to the cause of Pat Kehm's death. He attacked the integrity of Dr. Jacobs, telling the jury that his diagnosis was changed to TSS after I had contacted him and promised not to make a malpractice claim. He claimed that Jacobs had agreed to diagnose TSS in Pat Kehm in exchange for not being sued. He said the evidence pointed to the IUD being responsible and that a Tampax, not a Rely, was removed from Pat Kehm at the hospital the day she died.

P&G hit especially hard on the charge that the Kehms would be calling carpetbaggers from the East to prove their claim of product defect—an obvious reference to Dan and Tierno. The P&G attorney concluded that the company could not have grown to be the giant that it was if it did not do a good job of manufacturing safe and useful products like Crest toothpaste. Starr had remained in the courtroom after jury selection ended. At the noon recess, she told me that the P&G opening statement had been effective, that it had to be countered early in the evidence. Neither of us was aware that the points made in P&G's opening statement had been shaped by the reactions and comments of the jurors in the three Lincoln mock trials.

Coincidental with Bruce Dan's arrival in Cedar Rapids the night before the trial began, wet snow began to fall, and by morning, a one-foot blanket covered the ground. Dan had not brought a topcoat when he left balmy Atlanta, but although he was shivering when he arrived at the federal building to testify, he told Nan that the snow was a good omen. Since white is the symbol of purity and virtue—it meant good luck for our side, he said. Offhandedly, he told her that this was a Chinese way of looking at things. Later in the week, after Dan had left the stand, my wife told me she had encountered another good omen, this time in the form of baseball scores on the radio—Dan's home town of Atlanta had beaten Cincinnati.

As Dan entered the federal building, Starr, who was preparing to return to Des Moines, was introduced to him. One of her last acts before leaving was to tell the ex-CDC official that his mustache needed trimming. She didn't like the way it drooped downward around both corners of his mouth, saying it made him look sinister. Dan offered no objection as Starr took a pair of manicure scissors from her purse and

proceeded to trim the mustache back so that it remained
entirely above his upper lip. As a lawyer, I felt slightly embarrassed about the spectacle of altering a superficial appearance in order to conform to a preconceived idea of what
influences jurors. As we walked into the courtroom, I told
Dan that P&G hadn't waited until cross-examination to attack his fees. They had done so in the opening statement.
Dan smiled and shrugged his shoulders.

I began my examination of Dan by having him tell the
jury about his medical training and his employment and
general duties with the Centers for Disease Control from
1979 to 1981. I wanted the jury to know that Dan was no
lightweight despite his age. I asked questions that informed
the jury that Dan was board certified in internal medicine,
which meant three separate national board examinations,
three years residency training, being recommended by his
superiors and then a rigorous two-day examination. I also
brought to the jury's attention that Dan had over two dozen
articles published in medical and scientific journals and had
been awarded the Alex D. Langmuir Prize, conferred each
year for the outstanding manuscript on epidemiologic investigation and research done in preventing a major health
problem. Dan then detailed the history and purpose of the
CDC and his responsibility with the Epidemic Intelligence
Service of the CDC.

Next, Dan told the jury about the basic principles of infectious disease—how microorganisms cause illness by either direct damage to the body tissue or by releasing potent
toxins, how the body tries to protect itself from disease, how
some microorganisms are helpful and some are hurtful, and
that the body has several dozen or even hundreds of different species of bacteria in it any any one time. Dan explained
how the presence of bacteria in the nose, mouth or in the
case of women, in the vagina, does not usually make a person ill. Something has to happen for the *Staph aureus* in the
vagina to cause sickness in the woman.

Knowing that P&G would ask Dan about TSS in males and nonmenstruating women, and wanting to take the wind out of their sails, I asked Dan:

"Does Toxic Shock Syndrome affect only women?"

"No, sir. Anyone who has an infection with this particular bacteria is a potential risk for developing Toxic Shock Syndrome. We have seen this in men, in boys, in nonmenstruating women."

Anticipating the Yale expert, Feinstein's, attack on retrospective case control studies, I asked if such studies were unusual for the CDC's purposes. Dan said it was the main method of study for their work. When asked why, Dan answered:

"At the CDC, we cannot afford the time to spend years investigating certain diseases . . . the CDC's main mission is to prevent unnecessary disease and death. The way we do that very quickly is to do a quick retrospective study of looking at people who got the disease and people who did not, to find what was the critical factor, and hopefully eliminate the factor."

"In June of 1980, were people getting seriously sick and dying from Toxic Shock Syndrome?" I asked.

"Yes, sir."

There were seven epidemiological studies, Dan told the jury, two by the CDC and five by state public health agencies, and they all showed a significant association between tampons and TSS in menstruating women.

Dan told of meetings with P&G in the summer of 1980 and so I asked him:

"My client's wife died in September of 1980. In June, did your task force tell Procter & Gamble's representatives of your conclusions with respect to this association?"

"Yes, sir, many times."

Dan then told the jury he met with P&G people on August 15, 1980, three weeks before Pat Kehm's death, and told them that TSS was increasing at an accelerating rate, that there were more than three hundred validated cases and that the incidence was greater than originally estimated. I showed Dan a blowup of a P&G memo dated August 15, 1980:

"The CDC investigators are convinced that the use of tampons promotes and may even be necessary for the disease in those menstruating women who carry the organism and are susceptible."

"You told Procter & Gamble that?"

"Yes, sir."

"Do you still believe that today?"

"Most certainly."

"Did they issue any warning to their customers?"

"Not to my knowledge."

"Did they continue to aggressively promote on advertising on radio, on television, in the newspapers and magazines, urging people to use their product?"

"Yes, sir. I received a sample in my own mailbox at home."

"Free sample?"

"Yes, sir."

I then turned to a P&G memo of August 21, 1980. It was a report of data showing that about 36 percent of the TSS cases in Minnesota used Rely tampons.

"What is the significance of that from an epidemiologic standpoint?"

"It shows there is a disproportionate share of Toxic Shock Syndrome in menstruating women who use Rely tampons."

In a hushed voice I asked Dan:

"Pat Kehm was alive then. Did Procter & Gamble know about that disproportionate share of their product's involvement with Toxic Shock Syndrome?"

"Yes, sir, this is their memorandum."

"From their files?"

"Yes, sir."

I then turned to the CDC II study in September 1980, which sought to identify specific tampon brand involvement. In the CDC II, all the cases were recent TSS victims—those who had gotten ill in July and August 1980. By September, the CDC had enough recent TSS cases that they didn't have to reach back over a two-year period to come up with fifty TSS victims. Dan explained that the results of CDC II showed, again, that tampon usage occurred in 100 percent of all cases of TSS, and that Rely tampons were inordinately involved with much higher risk for development of TSS.

Then, I asked Dan the question about causation that we had discussed in Denver.

"Do tampons cause Toxic Shock Syndrome?"

"No."

At that point, P&G attorneys smiled, but not for long.

"Doctor, do tampons cause Toxic Shock Syndrome in menstruating women?"

"That's a different question and obviously the answer to that is yes."

"Do Rely tampons cause TSS in menstruating women?"

"Yes."

Dan told the jury that since a woman might be free of *Staph aureus* in her vagina one month but not the next month, all menstruating women are potentially at risk of getting TSS if they use tampons.

I asked Dan about the meeting with the FDA and P&G on September 16, 1980, when P&G was advised of the CDC II results that showed women using Rely were at much higher risk of getting TSS than with other brands. Dan told the jury that P&G asked the CDC not to mention Rely by name when the study was released.

"And they asked you not to mention that in connection with what?"

"The publication of the MMWR public release of information about that study."

"Do you believe the release of that publication saved lives?"

MR. WOODSIDE: "This is after the death of Mrs. Kehm and therefore irrelevant."

THE COURT: "Overruled. You may answer."

"Undoubtedly the release of this information prevented many cases of the disease and prevented many deaths."

I then turned to Pat Kehm's hospital records:

"Do you have an opinion as to the cause of Mrs. Kehm's death?"

"Yes."

"Tell this jury."

"Mrs. Kehm died from Toxic Shock Syndrome."

"How did she die?"

"She died of apparently cardiac arrest. Her heart stopped beating from it."

"If Pat Kehm had not used Rely tampons in September of 1980, would she be alive today?"

"I think if she had not used Rely tampons, she would not have gotten Toxic Shock Syndrome."

Now, nearly through with my examination, I showed a June 27, 1980, blowup of a P&G memo that told P&G's salesmen about TSS, its symptoms and its association with tampons. I asked Dan to read aloud a portion of the memo. A hush fell over the courtroom as the CDC physician read: "When calling on physicians, do not initiate discussion of TSS."

I then showed Dan a P&G memo of September 23, 1980, that recognized: "A great many M.D.'s remain ill-informed with respect to the identification and treatment of TSS." I concluded my examination of Dan by asking:

"Would it have helped in the summer of 1980, if the tampon manufacturers had added to your voice and others at

CDC, in spreading the word about Toxic Shock Syndrome in tampons?"

"Clearly, getting the Public Health's message out to the American woman would have prevented many cases of the illness."

"Were you trying to educate the medical community about Toxic Shock Syndrome?"

"To the best of our ability, yes."

"Was Procter & Gamble trying when they told their representatives not to bring up the subject?"

"I suspect not."

It was now P&G's turn to cross-examine Dan.

Although I had brought out Dan's fee of $3,000 on examination, Woodside got Dan to admit that he had consulted with 30 to 40 attorneys who represented TSS victims and that he charged $300 for each consultation.

Woodside attacked the way the CDC studies were carried out by having Dan admit that the task force didn't personally review the medical records of all the TSS victims in the studies but relied on the treating physicians reading them. Dan responded:

"Yes, sir. We couldn't afford to wait for records to be mailed to us. We talked to the physicians long distance on the phone while they had the medical records in front of them and went over the medical records with them to get the data quickly."

Woodside tried to get Dan to agree with P&G that Pat Kehm didn't have TSS because no doctor reported seeing the required rash.

"Like having a rash; you either got it or you don't, correct?"

"If it's noticed, yes."

Woodside got Dan to repeat that tampons, by themselves, don't cause TSS. Then he asked Dan:

"On the other hand, sir, the presence of toxigenic strain of Staphylococcus aureus can by itself cause Toxic Shock Syndrome in susceptible people, correct?"

"No, sir. Women who have the strain of bacteria in the vagina require the presence of a tampon to promote menstrually associated TSS."

When Dan ended an answer by saying that in June 1980 the CDC doctors were trying to find out as much as they could about this new disease, Woodside sarcastically commented:

"Sort of exciting, wasn't it?"

"Excuse me?" Dan responded, raising an eyebrow at the P&G attorney.

"You found it sort of exciting," Woodside shot back.

"I think all epidemiologists would find it interesting to try to find the cause of a disease, yes sir," Dan coolly replied.

Woodside casually made a reference to the date of the CDC II questionnaire. Mike Kehm caught my eye when Woodside did so. The questionnaire of the study that would ultimately drive Rely from the market and save an indeterminate number of lives was dated September 5, 1980—the date that Pat Kehm initially went to the Mercy Hospital emergency room, exactly one night before she died. Woodside intended to argue that if the CDC didn't know the cause of TSS on September 5, 1980, how could P&G? Woodside had Dan read from the questionnaire what the CDC interviewer would tell the TSS victims and controls:

"I am calling from the Center for Disease Control in Atlanta. We are studying Toxic Shock Syndrome, a disease of unknown cause that has received much publicity lately."

Woodside drove home his point.

"Now, therefore, as of September 5th, 1980, the cause of Toxic Shock Syndrome had not been proven, correct?"

But Dan threw off the challenge:

> "No, sir. That was what was read to the interviewees *not*
> to bias them. As you can see, the second paragraph says
> we are trying to determine the cause of this disease and
> any factors which may increase the risk of acquiring it.
> One doesn't want to pre-bias an interviewee by telling
> them we *understand* the cause and want to ask you certain
> factors. This study was looking specifically at tampon use
> and tampon brands. You will notice we didn't mention
> tampons or tampon brands in the introduction to the cases."

This would be helpful when the P&G expert from Yale
would testify to claim that the CDC studies were biased against
tampons.

Woodside pressed P&G's complaint that publicity about
tampons and TSS would have biased the outcome of CDC II.
Dan used a refinement of the winner's argument, when the
losing team complained that muddy playing conditions affected the outcome, that: "It rained on both sides of the field."
He told the jury:

> "There was no reason to suspect that people who hap-
> pened to have had a disease would be any more likely to
> have watched Walter Cronkite or read a newspaper than
> those women who used tampons, were menstruating, but
> had not gotten sick. There was no bias there. The public-
> ity was assumed to be equal for both groups."

When Woodside continued to suggest TSS victims would
claim they used Rely because of publicity, Dan calmly replied:

> "She had every reason to tell us the truth, and we asked
> her to go to her closet, bring back the box of tampons she
> was using and read to us exactly what it said. Now, there
> was no reason I can think of why watching publicity about
> tampons on TV would make a woman change the name
> of her brand specifically when we said we had not found
> any difference in brands.

Woodside then challenged the CDC studies, arguing that vaginal cultures had not been done to see if the cases and the controls had the same strains of *Staphylococcus aureus* present.

> "I think if you wanted to make the perfect study, which you could do at your leisure, and that public health and public lives were not at stake, you would gather together women who have toxic shock and go out and gather many people who have the same staph in the vagina and do the same study. Perfect studies were not our mission. Our mission was to save lives, not to make perfect studies."
> "And just to make it clear, CDC I or CDC II were not perfect studies?"
> "I don't think there has ever been a perfect study."
> "If there has, you have not done one, have you?"
> "No, sir."

Woodside also got Dan to concede that it was not until after Pat Kehm had died that the specific association with Rely tampons had been established, although Dan claimed that it had been suspected from the early results of the Utah I study in June of 1980. Woodside also called the jury's attention to the fact that the FDA Bureau of Medical Devices had reservations about CDC I and the CDC's claim of a tampon association in June of 1980.

> "In that article Mr. Sava is criticizing CDC for having an inadequate study design. Is that correct?"
> "No. I don't think there is any criticism. It says it has reservations on how the development of TSS is related to tampons."

A little humor crept in when Woodside asked Dan about a senate subcommittee hearing chaired by Senator Ted Kennedy on June 6, 1980. The subcommittee was investigating toxic waste dumps, like the Love Canal. A senate staff member saw the May 27, 1980, *MMWR* about Toxic Shock Syndrome and, thinking it might be related to the subject of toxic dumps, called Drs. Foege and Shands to Washington to testify at the hearing. Woodside inquired:

"The toxic dump and Love Canal doesn't have anything to do with Toxic Shock Syndrome, is that correct?"

"Unless you know something I don't," Dan responded.

It was at that hearing that Dr. Foege, assistant surgeon general and director of the CDC, had told the senators that he expected the mystery of TSS would be solved by Christmas of that year. Dan claimed that he said it in a joking manner. P&G claimed that Foege had gone out on a limb in his prediction, and CDC I and II were hurriedly thrown together in order to meet the Foege-imposed deadline. Dan denied it.

Woodside then showed Dan a letter written by Shands on August 19, 1980, in which she stated that, "Tampons are not the most probable cause of TSS in young women." Dan agreed that was what Shands said, but he speculated that the statement was in response to whether tampons, alone, cause TSS and they do not.

Woodside then asked the court if the lawyers could approach the bench so he could make a request outside the presence of the jury.

With the jury excused, Woodside told McManus that P&G had a videotape of a T.V. interview given by Dan on a New York television station on August 28, 1980, and he wished to show it to the jury to impeach Dan's testimony on direct examination that he had said, back in August 1980, that tampons are necessary to cause TSS in menstruating women.

I asked Woodside how long P&G had the tape. The P&G attorney responded that it had been flown in on a special plane at 10:00 the previous night. I objected because the videotape was a type of physical evidence that the court wanted shown to opposing counsel in advance of trial. Woodside countered that P&G didn't know Dan was going to testify that he had publicly stated in August 1980 that tampons are necessary to cause TSS in menstruating women. The court, after reviewing the tape while the jury was excused, granted permission to Woodside to show it and to question Dan about it. The videotape began with a television reporter saying, "Dr. Bruce Dan of the CDC explains": Then Dan was shown on camera saying:

> "It is not a causal factor. It is associated with the use of tampons. In a sense menstruation doesn't cause the disease but it certainly is associated with it. There must be some factor necessary there for menstruation to make the disease happen. The disease is caused in that sense, by a toxin from a bacteria. There must be other factors that help this along. It is a very infrequent and rare disease and therefore it has to have a joining of several factors that come together to make the disease happen. One of them may be the fact that tampons in menstruating women make this happen. Men and children have this disease, obviously don't wear tampons. The disease is caused by the bacteria."

I began redirect examination of Dan by going directly to the videotape of his interview.

> "I got the impression watching that for the first time that you were in the middle of a sentence when you came on the screen. Did you get that impression?"
> "I can't remember all that went on but that obviously wasn't the beginning of the interview."
> "Do you know who spliced that?"
> "I have no idea."

Under questioning, Woodside admitted that the copy of the tape had come to him from P&G and not directly from the television station. I had Dan explain what he was saying in the television interview:

> "In the case of an abscess you don't need a tampon. As in the vagina, normally in a place of closed infection, you need a tampon in associated cases. Not the only factor.

The tampon, bacteria, menstruation, cause toxic shock. You need them all together."

"And you told Procter & Gamble that, did you not, in August of 1980, and in July of 1980, and in June of 1980?"

"We told everyone that, scientists, media and everyone."

I referred to the situation of mosquitos and malaria to draw an analogy to tampons.

"So technically speaking, do mosquitos cause malaria?"

"Mosquitos themselves don't cause malaria. Obviously, you have to have the mosquito carrying the malaria parasite. You need several things. Susceptible person, you need the mosquito, and the malaria parasite. Some people are immune."

"Something then enters the body in the case of malaria and causes the disease that is known as malaria."

"Right. The prevention of malaria did not wipe out the parasite. You wipe out the mosquito that triggers the event and you wipe out malaria."

"And that was done by the CDC?"

"Yes, twenty, thirty years ago."

Then I had Dan read the rest of Dr. Shands's letter, not just the excerpt Woodside mentioned:

"It is also possible that once in the vagina the tampon may promote growth of the organism or elaboration of a toxin. But the tampon itself, unlike cigarettes and saccharin products, does not represent a risk to a woman in the absence of the Staph. aureus organism."

I concluded my redirect examination by introducing a blowup of the P&G memo I had received from Wichita lawyer Mark Hutton. After having Dan tell the jury that teenagers were most susceptible to TSS, I asked Dan to read aloud how P&G, despite its knowledge of the reported tampon association with TSS, was planning in late August 1980 to encourage "tampon use, and especially Rely use, by young women." Dan read from the P&G memo dated August 27, 1980, which told of a P&G study conducted among family physicians and pediatricians to determine whether P&G could build an aggressive level of support for Rely with those doctors. I then interrupted Dan to ask:

> "What type of age patient does a pediatrician treat?"
>
> "Generally young children and adolescents."
>
> "Would you read the next paragraph, please?"
>
> "A major objective is to encourage tampon use, and especially Rely use, by young women. . . . We therefore turned to the family physician and pediatrician medical audiences as the only remaining opportunity to utilize the known impact of the health care profession to stimulate positive results for Rely . . . It appears that we have several school program opportunities that will provide the broad reach and high impact we are looking for."

Reporters were straining to read the blowup describing P&G's efforts to convert young girls—those most susceptible to TSS—to Rely. What made the memo shocking was the fact that it was written more than two months after P&G had been told of the tampon association, and three weeks after the first lawsuit against P&G.

Dan had made an excellent witness and got our case off to a good start, I felt. The next witness, family practitioner John Jacobs, followed Dan in the witness box. It was vital that I destroy the claim P&G made in the opening statement that I had talked Jacobs into changing the cause of Pat Kehm's death. Not only did that impugn both our reputations, but it was untrue. And Jacobs and I weren't the only persons in that courtroom who knew it was a lie.

Roland Kreckler, a *Cedar Rapids Gazette* reporter covering the trial, told me after the P&G opening statement that he remembered a *Gazette* story quoting Jacobs as having publicly stated that Pat Kehm died of TSS, and he thought it had occurred soon after her death and before the date that I had first contacted Jacobs. Kreckler's recall was correct, and I was able to use the *Gazette* story of September 24, as irrefutable proof that P&G had made an unfounded personal attack on Jacobs and myself.

> "Were you aware that that charge had been made in this courtroom?"
>
> "I first heard it on the news last night and I read it again this morning in the *Cedar Rapids Gazette*."

I asked whether the charge was true. The court overruled P&G's objection to the question, and Jacobs answered:

> "It was false. I did not change the diagnosis."

I handed Jacobs the death certificate that had been signed on September 19, 1980, which stated the cause of death was toxic shock secondary to staph colonization of the cervix and uterus.

> "In other words, Doctor, ten days before you and I had even discussed this subject you had made the diagnosis of Toxic Shock Syndrome on the official records required to be filed with the State Department of Health for the State of Iowa?"
>
> "Yes."
>
> "And before we talked on the 29th day of September, 1980, was there not a report in the *Cedar Rapids Gazette* reporting on your diagnosis of Toxic Shock Syndrome for Patricia Kehm?"
>
> "I believe that it is correct, it was before our conversation."

Jacobs's further testimony outlined how he and the others had tried to save Pat Kehm's life. Jacobs explained how his initial diagnosis of TSS versus septic shock was what doctors call a differential diagnosis, meaning that doctors list the different possible diagnoses until they have all the medical evidence. In Pat Kehm's case, the additional evidence was the lab reports on blood testing and culturing for bacteria. When the lab reports came back, the diagnosis of septic shock was ruled out while TSS was confirmed.

> "Would it have been possible for you—would it have been proper medicine for you to have reached a final diagnosis without those laboratory tests?"
>
> "I would consider it improper."

On cross-examination, Jacobs showed resentment at P&G's attempt at character assassination. He did agree he was not an expert on tampons and that until he treated Pat Kehm on September 6, 1980, he had heard and knew little about TSS.

P&G then attempted to shift the blame for Pat's death to the emergency room physician who saw her the night before she died.

> "Let me ask you this: Based on this record, had you been the physician, was Mrs. Kehm savable at this point?"
>
> "It certainly would appear so. I would say yes, but I can't prove that without further information."

P&G then got Jacobs to admit that the tampon was discarded without thought being given to testing or culturing it despite the fact Quetsch had mentioned to Jacobs the possibility of Pat Kehm having tampon-related TSS.

> "Was it contrary to hospital policy to have disposed of that tampon when it might be the center of your focus and in what you were looking for?"
>
> "I really don't know what hospital policy would be on that."
>
> "Well, I understand that if a woman comes in with a hangnail you probably aren't going to save the tampon, but if she came in with what was thought to be toxic shock and you believed it to be associated somehow with tampons, would it have been a good idea to save the tampon?"

"Well, I think—I certainly would have saved it had I known a year and a half later we were in court over it. At the time, as I told you, I was more concerned about saving that lady's life than going to court."

P&G pressed Jacobs on the failure to save and culture the tampon while the IUD was saved and cultured, implying that Jacobs really suspected the IUD and not the tampon.

"In view of the fact that the tampon was thrown away and disposed of, there is no way that we can show whether or not that tampon had, and prove that that tampon had, any bacteria in it, can we, from a clinical point of view?"
"No."

Then P&G's attorney asked Jacobs about his conversation with me on September 29, 1980. Jacobs was asked to read the note he dictated about the call.

"He assured me that Mr. Kehm had no animosity or doubts concerning the medical care, either from the attending physician or from the hospital employee's standpoint, and was not interested in pursuing any legal course against either one."
"Now, when you say 'either one' or 'not interested in pursuing a legal course against either one,' are you referring to yourself and the hospital?"
"That's what my recollection would be, yes."
"And this is the same hospital that you were president of the staff of at that time, right?"
"For whatever that's worth, yes."

P&G was particularly interested in Jacobs's last note: "We did not talk about the IUD."

Jacobs was asked why he made the reference to the IUD in his notes, implying that Jacobs must have thought the IUD had a role to play in Pat Kehm's illness.

"Well, did you think it was peculiar that that was not discussed by Mr. Riley and you during that conversation?"

"At that point I would have to say I don't know and didn't know what Mr. Riley's level of sophistication about medical contraceptive devices was and whether he would have talked about it or not. I don't know why he didn't ask about it."

"But you were concerned that that had not been mentioned, and you memorialized it, did you not?"

"I made a statement it wasn't talked about."

The court sustained my objection to a question asking Jacobs if he notified his malpractice carrier of a possible claim on the case.

The cross-examination of Jacobs ended with the doctor admitting that he did not know how tampons caused TSS, that the problem was still under examination and that he was not a research scientist.

On redirect examination, I established that Jacobs's lack of knowledge of exactly how tampons caused TSS would not change his opinion that Pat Kehm died of tampon related TSS. Jacobs also told the jury he felt the IUD picked up the *Staph aureus* when it was pulled through the vagina at its removal.

I continued to bring the jurors' attention back to the P&G memo that I contended showed that P&G was trying to "let sleeping dogs lie" when it told P&G sales representatives not to initiate discussion about TSS when calling on M.D.s. I reminded Jacobs of an answer on cross-examination that Pat Kehm was savable when she went to the emergency room the night before she died.

"Did Procter & Gamble ever notify you, as a doctor, during the summer of 1980, that a product that it was promoting over television and in the newspapers had been associated with a sometimes fatal illness?"

"No."

I ended his redirect examination by having Jacobs read the instructions on the P&G memo that P&G employees should not initiate disclosure of TSS and then asked the family practitioner:

> "Would it have helped, in your opinion, as a doctor of many years, if this large company with its great resources had helped disseminate information about their product in connection with the risk associated with it to even a fraction of the extent to which they advertise the sale of that product on radio, television, and in the newspapers?"
>
> "Certainly would have helped."

On that note, I ended his redirect examination and Jacobs stepped down from the witness stand. As the doctor walked past Mike Kehm, he touched his hand reassuringly to the young man's shoulder.

13

"*Yes, I believe that the tampon creates those microbiological conditions necessary for the elaboration of the Staphylococcus aureus, more so than any tampon on the market.*"

Testimony of microbiologist Tierno on cross-examination

Jacobs had been on the stand for part of Tuesday, April 6, the second day of trial, and for most of Wednesday, the 7th of April. After that much scientific and technical information from Dan and Jacobs, I felt it would be a good idea to give the jury some relief. So I called as my next witness, Sue Myers, the twenty-five-year-old Omaha wife and mother. She told the jury how she had never had trouble with her menstrual periods until she used Rely during her cycles of September and October of 1979. She described her near death experience the first time she developed TSS and her realization when she developed the same symptoms during the next period that the only thing common to both incidents was her use of Rely tampons. She told of how she contacted P&G, how she was told that Rely was made of things like rayon and cotton. She explained her reaction to that to the jury:

"And I thought well, geez, there has got to be something else, you know. This just isn't right."

"Have you ever had any trouble with cotton and rayon before?"

"No, never at all. I never had any trouble with any kind of tampon."

I handed Myers a P&G memo of June 27, 1980, advising company personnel of the CDC I Study that had found an association between tampons and TSS. The memo instructed P&G personnel not to quote from the study unless someone asked specific questions. The memo listed questions. One of those questions was whether P&G had ever received any complaints of severe illness or reaction to Rely. Since Myers had complained to P&G that Rely caused her a near death illness in 1979, I asked her to read P&G's prepared statement to the news media and public dated June 27, 1980.

"In all our extensive testing and market experience with Rely, we have never been aware of any severe illness or reaction caused by the use of our product."

P&G's cross-examination centered on the failure of Myers to complete a lengthy questionnaire that P&G had sent her following her complaint. The witness explained that the reason she called P&G was to find out what Rely was made of so she could avoid the same components in other products. She did not realize that filling out the questionnaire might help others because she thought she had a unique allergy. When she read an article in the *Omaha World Herald* nine months later, she suddenly became aware that other women were experiencing the same illness. Had P&G followed up on her inquiry about the components in Rely by explaining to her of the importance of the questionnaire and how it might help others, instead of telling her on the telephone that the product was safe and made of cotton and rayon, she told P&G's attorney that she would have happily filled out P&G's form.

When Mercy Hospital nurse Lois Sterenchuk took the stand, she told the jury that in the frenzy accompanying the life-saving efforts and the notating of those efforts in the hospital charts, she had used the generic term "Tampax" to refer to the tampon she had removed from Pat Kehm in the emergency room. Sterenchuk testified that she referred to all tampons as Tampax and all sanitary napkins as Kotex, because those were the brands that had first been marketed and the only ones with which she was personally familiar.

I asked the nurse to immerse a Rely and a Tampax in a glass of water. At that point McManus asked me:

> "What is the need of putting it in the water?"
>
> "Because, Your Honor, they look quite a bit different when they are actually in an expanded form. Is that not true?"
>
> "That is right," Sterenchuk responded.
>
> "You mean a Tampax looks different than a Rely when they are wet?" McManus asked.
>
> "All the difference in the world, Your Honor."

After the tampons had swollen, they no longer resembled the cylinder shape they do when dry. I asked the nurse which looked like the one she removed from Pat Kehm. She unhesitantly pointed to the Rely tampon.

On cross-examination, the P&G attorney asked Sterenchuk about a drawing of the tampon that she had made during a deposition. Her drawing resembled a bell with a string extending from the top of the bell. Pat Kehm had used Playtex tampons before switching to Rely for her September 1980 period. The P&G lawyer immersed a Playtex tampon in a glass of water and held it by the string so that the tampon hung downward. Held in that fashion, it somewhat resembled the drawing that Sterenchuk had made at the deposition. However, unlike the tea-bag-type construction of a Rely tampon, the Playtex tampon consisted of a number of square-shaped patches of clothlike material sewn together at one end where the string attaches. Held upside down, the wet patches of cloth clung together and resembled the shape of her deposition drawing.

But nurse Sterenchuk wasn't going to let the P&G attorney mislead the jury. She acknowledged that when held in that position, there was a resemblance between their shapes, but she pointed out that she hadn't held the tampon in that manner when she held it up in the emergency room, and she asked to be handed the wet Playtex tampon. As the jury watched her intently, she turned the tampon upright, pointing out that that was the way she held it in the emergency room. As she did so, the square patches of the Playtex tampon collapsed around her fingers and ended any resemblance to the bell-shaped tampon Sterenchuk had drawn at her deposition.

The P&G attorney recovered enough to get the nurse to agree with Jacobs that it would have been better if she had not discarded the tampon so that it could have been cultured. He also got Sterenchuk to acknowledge that she had not observed a rash on Pat Kehm's body. On redirect examination, Sterenchuk told the jury that she was unaware when she removed the tampon that tampons were associated with TSS.

At this point, I felt our case was convincing that Pat died of TSS from using Rely. The only question left, I felt, was how Rely tampons caused TSS in menstruating women. I hoped that my next witness, Dr. Tierno, would supply that answer. Tierno had conducted extensive research since his deposition so I decided to take a chance on his demeanor on the witness stand and asked him to testify in person.

As he began his testimony, Tierno told the jury how his wife, Josephine, had initiated his interest in the subject of TSS. P&G's attorneys and legal assistants snickered when Tierno told of taking a culture from his wife and explaining to her that she had not gotten TSS using superabsorbent tampons because she had no *Staphylococcus aureus* present.

Tierno then described dissecting a Rely tampon and his observations about what happened to the little chips of CMC when immersed in water. He told the jury how the CMC swelled into a jellylike substance and cited scientific articles that had discussed how gelatinlike substances enhanced the production of toxins by *Staphylococcus aureus*, the bacterium associated with TSS.

> "And then I started to think about the gelling effect. The entire tampon when immersed in water gels. When it becomes profused with blood, it becomes analogous to a Petri dish of blood agar, which is what we use to grow bacteria on."
> "You mean to say that the tampon resembled a medium or liquid that is used to grow bacteria?"
> "A semisolid agar, yes, it did."

Tierno told the jury how he had written a letter to P&G and the FDA in October 1980, setting forth his opinion as to how Rely tampons increased the risk of TSS. Shortly afterwards, P&G microbiologist, James Widder, contacted Tierno and offered him a P&G grant. Tierno told Widder he hadn't the time to pursue the TSS inquiry further. When he renewed his interest in TSS the following year, P&G renewed its offer of grants and Tierno again turned them down.

I knew that P&G hoped to persuade the jury that Tierno was a kook and his theories no better. I intended to argue that P&G wouldn't be funding just anyone, therefore, P&G either felt he was knowledgeable or they were trying to silence him with their money.

Tierno emphasized that many factors are involved in the development of TSS in menstruating women. Not only was the vagina an ideal culture medium during menstruation, but the polyester foam and CMC chips provided a perfect environment for the growth of any *Staph aureus* and created a walled-off effect similar to an abscess. Acknowledging that TSS can occur naturally, Tierno testified that tampons created an artificial abscess in the vagina.

Tierno contended that one reason Rely was defective was

that the little chips of CMC were a food for bacteria, including *Staph aureus*. Enzymes broke down the synthetic cellulose. The court permitted Tierno to demonstrate how beta-glucosidase, an enzyme produced by bacteria that is known to inhabit the vagina, would break down the CMC absorbency chips in Rely. Placing several of the chips within a small, short vial, Tierno added a few drops of beta-glucosidase. Tierno predicted that the chips would be dissolved from the solid state in less than two hours since the enzyme action would be slowed by the cooler temperature of the courtroom compared to the body temperature within the human vagina. The vial was then given to the deputy clerk for safekeeping, and the court adjourned for the noon recess. When the vial was produced two hours later, the chips were nowhere to be seen. In their place was a slightly yellowish free-moving liquid.

We knew that P&G would contend that the fact that CMC could be used as a food for bacteria was immaterial since there would be plenty of food for bacteria in the vagina during menstruation whether or not a tampon was present—as if adding some CMC chips would have the same effect that throwing a bucket of water would have on the level of a lake. Tierno anticipated this by pointing out that there is not all that much blood flowing during a period (approximately one ounce over a four- to five-day time frame) and that it often flows intermittently. The presence of CMC would provide a continuous food supply to bacteria—something vital to their growth and toxin production.

Tierno said his laboratory tests showed that Rely carboxymethylcellulose was a food for bacteria in the vagina. I asked Tierno if it had been known in scientific literature for some time that a carboxymethylcellulose would break down under bacterial action. When Tierno agreed, he was asked when was the earliest time that such knowledge was available.

"There were articles in the 1920s, and, of course, in the forties and fifties and sixties."

"So a manufacturer of a tampon that was to use a substance such as carboxymethylcellulose would certainly have
had access to information of that kind in the scientific
literature?"

"Yes, sir."

Tierno then expressed his initial surprise about the results
of his experiments with Rely because he considered that any
product that is put in the vagina or any orifice that has normal
flora should be inert, and, in fact, he discovered it was not
inert but biodegradable, or able to be broken down.

I asked Tierno about tests that he had done on protein production by *Staph aureus* in the presence of Rely. Tierno pointed
out that exotoxins produced by bacteria are proteins, and that
he had conducted simple tests to measure the effect of Rely
tampons on inducing protein production. He told the jury the
Rely had caused *Staph aureus* to produce 21 percent more protein than in a similar broth without Rely.

"Is there any reason, Dr. Tierno, that a qualified microbiologist could not have performed the same test on Rely
components, and I am referring to protein production of
Staphylococcus aureus, before Rely was put on the market on a limited basis in 1974?"

"Anyone could have done what I did who is qualified
in microbiology."

"Were such tests feasible and practical in 1974?"

"Yes, sir."

"If Procter & Gamble did the testing and was aware of
the results, would that have been good or bad microbiological practice, Dr. Tierno?"

"Yes, if they knew of the results it would have been
bad to add a product like that knowingly."

"Would it also have been bad not to do that testing?"

"Of course that's the most basic and simple test. That's
the first test that should have been done."

I then offered into evidence the P&G memo dated September 12, 1980, that revealed P&G had obtained permission to export a modified Rely to Japan—one without carboxymethylcellulose.

I then asked Tierno the ultimate question.

> "Now, as a result of your research and based upon a reasonable degree of scientific and microbiological probability, do you have an opinion as to the relationship between Rely tampons and Toxic Shock Syndrome in menstruating women?"

Despite Woodside's objection to Tierno stating a medical opinion, the court allowed the microbiologist to answer.

> "Yes, I believe that the tampon creates those microbiological conditions necessary for the elaboration of the Staphylococcus aureus, more so than any tampon on the market."

On cross-examination, Woodside got Tierno to admit that he had not demonstrated the proteins produced by *Staph aureus* in the presence of Rely to be toxic. Woodside went on to suggest that the *Staph aureus* TSS toxin was a mutant strain that could not be predicted in advance. He used the wrong analogy with Tierno.

> "It is kind of like with a new car. We know that there is going to be a new model every year but we really don't know exactly what the new model is going to be. Is that a fair analogy?"
>
> "I can get that information on occasion. You can go to a dealer and they may show you what is on the drawing board."
>
> "Let me just— That is right. I agree with that," Woodside floundered.
>
> "Thank you, Dr. Woodside," Tierno said with an impish grin.

Tierno began to get the flavor of the courtroom atmosphere

and demonstrated it when Woodside asked him about *Staph
aureus* in women:

> "Now, you indicated that somewhere around ten or fif-
> teen percent of the women have Staphylococcus aureus
> in their vagina as part of their normal vaginal flora. Cor-
> rect?"
>
> "No. I said between five and fifteen percent, but, you
> know, we don't want to be picky."

Woodside then tried to put the blame on the women who
got TSS, pointing out that they were a relatively small percentage of women who were lacking in antibodies to fight the
toxin. Tierno wouldn't agree with that argument.

> "I agree with you that they are in a much higher risk. But
> the bottom line is in the insertion of the tampon and the
> proliferation of the organism."

Woodside did score a point when Tierno became defensive
about the fees that he charged P&G in connection with a deposition in the Lampshire case.

> "Do you recall that for taking your deposition you charged
> me the sum of $5,750?"
>
> "I appeared for two days in deposition."
>
> THE COURT: "Answer the question."
>
> "It is true, and it is an undercharge for what I had to
> go through," Tierno answered.

Tierno was still chafing over what had been an exhausting
eighteen-hour videotaped deposition, which he had found hu-
miliating because of the scope of the inquiry. The questions
put to him by Woodside had covered his entire lifetime and
included irrelevant and personal questions regarding child-
hood and school events. Tierno had gotten a measure of satisfaction by charging $250 an hour for deposition time and
then using the money to finance his TSS research. He had
turned down offers of direct funding in order to keep his independence as a scientist. I had been struck by the irony that

every time a tampon company subjected Tierno to a deposition (he eventually was deposed more than forty times), the tampon companies were providing him with money he used for research to prove the tampon and TSS connection. Thus, Tierno, and his colleague Bruce Hanna, got tampon company funding without any restriction or loss of their independence.

Having recently taken Tierno's deposition in another Rely case, Woodside knew about an experiment that Tierno had done testing a Rely tampon in a human vagina. Woodside sought to put Tierno in a bad light for causing risk to the person and, if that failed, to embarrass Tierno by having him identify who the volunteer was.

> "As I understand it, you did have experimental work done on your wife, didn't you?"
> "I never testified as to in whom it was done."
> "But, in fact, it was your wife?"
> "I have no qualms about mentioning it."

Woodside ended his cross-examination by pointing out that the CDC did not ask Tierno to give any presentation after they received his open letter of October 10, 1980. Tierno replied that that was correct—that the CDC advised him to pursue it on his own and publish it, which he had done.

To ensure that the jury understood that Mrs. Tierno was at no risk in participating in her husband's experiment, and to contrast that with unsuspecting purchasers of Rely like Pat Kehm, I had Tierno explain, on redirect examination, that Mrs. Tierno couldn't get TSS because she didn't carry *Staph aureus*. Indicating that Mrs. Tierno was present in the courtroom, I asked:

> "And she knew what you were asking her to experiment in doing did she not?"
> "Yes."
> "She knew before she put the Rely tampon in that there were not Staphylococcus aureus present, did she?"
> "Yes."

"Was that true of many women in America who received free Rely samples in the mail or were urged by advertisements to purchase Rely tampons? Did they know whether or not they had Staphylococcus aureus in their vagina?"

"No."

McManus adjourned court following Tierno's testimony. As we left the courtroom, Tierno and I were joined by our wives and two TSS plaintiffs' lawyers from out of state. The other lawyers had no emotional involvement in the case other than the natural desire to see P&G lose. They remarked that Tierno had done a good job overall providing the jury with a scientific explanation for the relationship of tampons and TSS.

Our talk turned to P&G's army of legal help. I told how P&G had ordered transcripts—"dailies"—of each day's testimony so that they would get the morning testimony by 1:00 p.m. that same day and the afternoon testimony by 5:30 p.m. that night. That alone would cost more than $25,000. If we had ordered dailies, the cost would have been split in half by both sides, but since my client could not afford even $12,500, P&G ordered the dailies for their exclusive use and paid the full price. One of the visiting plaintiff's attorneys remarked that having dailies would just add extra work. "It's not a pain if you've got ten other attorneys and legal assistants to go through them looking for bits of gold or rust depending on your point of view," the other attorney answered.

I expressed the view that the dailies were invaluable to P&G because it allowed them to circumvent McManus's rule excluding witnesses from the courtroom. While our witnesses couldn't hear what the other witnesses on either side said and, technically, neither could theirs, P&G's witnesses could read all the testimony and create their own instant replays by simply going back and rereading whatever they had an interest in. They could modify their testimony to comport with what their fellow witnesses had said, and they could see the approaches that I had been taking on cross-examination and be ready for them. Tierno broke in to tell me not to worry, there was still only one truth.

After Tierno and his wife left for the airport, I asked the other lawyers if they intended to ask him to testify at their cases. I recall one of them answering, "Let's see how the case comes out. Then we can decide."

14

". . . they let my wife die, and, as I understand it, punitive damages are to punish."

Testimony of Mike Kehm regarding the reason for his claim.

As the fifth day of trial began, I called Dr. Richard Quetsch to the stand. I let the jury know that Quetsch served his residency in internal medicine at the Mayo Clinic just in case McManus granted P&G's request to let the Mayo doctors, who had issued the Rely press release, testify.

Quetsch told about the mild case of TSS he had seen a few weeks before Mrs. Kehm's illness so "I guess my mind was more alert to the possibility. There really aren't too many things that cause shock in young women that age," he explained to the jury. Thanks to the FDA bulletin and the extreme mildness of that earlier case, Quetsch had been able to save one woman's life. I thought if only the emergency room physician had seen the FDA bulletin, or if only P&G had not kept the lid on, Pat Kehm would be alive and the young man sitting next to me wouldn't be nervously straightening, loosening and retightening his tie and pulling on the cuffs of his shirt.

Quetsch told the jury that the entry in the hospital records to the effect that the doctors were unable to establish whether

Pat was using a tampon was written right after Pat died and before they learned a tampon had been removed.

> "But you have no doubt that a tampon was removed, because it appears in the nurses' charts?"
>
> "When Mrs. Sterenchuk says something, I believe it," Quetsch said emphatically.

Quetsch concluded his testimony with the opinion that the tampon was an important factor in Pat's death.

On cross-examination, Woodside asked how Quetsch could now testify that tampons were a factor in Pat Kehm's death when he did not know whether or not she had a tampon in place at the time. But Quetsch had an answer for the P&G attorney:

> "There's no law about Toxic Shock Syndrome or the use of tampons that says she had to be still wearing it when she came to the emergency room. She could well have had the illness and the tampon had been removed at home because her period was ending or for some other reason."

Woodside hammered at the fact that Quetsch had thought Pat had TSS when he not only didn't know she had been wearing a tampon at the hospital, but didn't know if she ever used them.

Again, Quetsch had a logical answer for Woodside.

> "I did not know that she had not been, and since the illness was so characteristic of the illness caused by tampons, it was reasonable for me to assume that she had indeed been using them, whether or not one was found at that time or not."
>
> "And that was just an assumption you were making, correct?"
>
> "A very reasonable assumption," Quetsch concluded.

The next witness may have been the greatest victim of Pat Kehm's illness and death—maybe an even greater victim than

Pat, herself. Colleen Jones had repeatedly urged her sister to try Rely—and Colleen would never forgive herself.

She told the jury about the happy and loving marriage of her sister and Mike Kehm.

> "They were kind to each other all the time and thoughtful, and when Pat had the kids, he would always send up roses, and she would knit him sweaters and a neckscarf, and they loved each other very much."
>
> "What about downgrading each other and things like that?"
>
> "I have never heard them bad talk each other."
>
> "How did they spend their spare time?"
>
> "Oh, I know they would go out, and they would go dancing, and they would go on picnics, and they would come out and visit us when we were camping, and I know once Patty even drug Mike to a disco lesson."

Colleen smiled faintly as she spoke and Mike smiled too, lowering his head and shaking it slowly as he remembered that night. It was only an instant between questions, a shared family joke, but that night was once again vivid to Mike and Colleen even now. Watching them, we all were reminded that Pat had been a real person—not just a picture in a newspaper story from the past.

> "How close were you to Pat?"
>
> "I was very close."

Lowering my voice, I asked:

> "How did your sister come to use Rely tampons?"

Looking down at her hands, she answered:

> "I told her to try them."

In the most emotionally charged scene of the trial, McManus, over the vehement objections of the P&G attorneys, allowed Colleen to read her sister's last diary entries of August 25 and 29, 1980. Crying softly at times, she read:

"Katie was baptized yesterday. Colleen and Terry were the sponsors."

Colleen smiled slightly through her tears at her sister's comment about how Andrea had looked after playing at Colleen's house.

"She was a real good girl. She is drooling a lot. Might be teething. Andrea got filthy dirty at Colleen's today. She must have had a good time. . . . I love our little family."

Absolute quiet fell over the courtroom as she proceeded to read the August 29, 1980 entry—written just eight days before Pat's death.

Colleen then told the jury how she started using Rely tampons after both her mother and mother-in-law got free samples in the mail and had given them to her sometime in the winter of 1979–80. I asked if she had thought it was a fine product and she said yes.

"Made by a responsible company?"
"Yes."
"Whose many products you had probably used without any problems in the past?"
"I used to."
"You mean you are conducting a one-woman boycott right now?"

An objection was sustained, so I changed my question:

"In any event, when you said you used to, the point is up until your sister's death you used many Procter & Gamble products?"
"Yes, I did."

Colleen then told of visiting her sister two days before she died. Pat was lying on the couch and said she wasn't feeling well. She remembers asking Pat if she had tried Rely yet.

"And what did she say?"
"She said 'I am using them now.'"

"Did she say how she liked them?"

"She said, 'I have been feeling so bad that I haven't noticed.'"

She told about rushing to the hospital when she learned that her sister had been taken there by ambulance. When asked what she observed on arrival, she testified:

"Well, Michael was there, and he was real scared, I could tell. And he said they had Pat in the other room cutting down her legs to try to put IVs in them."

"You did not have an opportunity to see Pat at that time?"

"I didn't want to see her."

"Why is that?"

"I was upset and I didn't want her to see me upset, because I know if she seen me upset that she would be—"

"More frightened?"

"Yes."

I ended my direct examination by having Colleen explain that she was caring for Mike's two little girls, Andrea and Katie, during the weekdays while Mike worked and that Mike had them on the weekend.

"You are doing what any sister would do under the circumstances?"

"Yes."

P&G's goal on cross-examination was to suggest that Pat Kehm might have been using her former tampon brand preference, Playtex, during part of her September menstrual period—leftovers from her August period. Colleen had to concede she didn't know the answer and that it was possible. Colleen also admitted that she had not seen a rash on Pat when she picked up Andrea to care for her on Friday morning, September 5, but she explained that Pat was bundled up in her bed and the bedroom was dark. The P&G attorney pressed:

"Well, the answer is you didn't see any rash, for whatever reason, isn't that right?"

Colleen agreed that she had not.

Seeking to show indifference on Mike's part to his children, he asked Colleen if Mike saw them only on weekends. Colleen replied:

"No, he visits about three evenings during the week."

On redirect examination, Colleen testified that it was the best arrangement for her to look after the kids during the week while Mike worked. Earlier, P&G had gotten Colleen to mention that her brother-in-law paid her $250 per month.

"Is there any place in town that Mike could obtain the services that you provide those little girls for anywhere near that sum of money?" I asked.

"I don't think so," she replied.

Jean Robinson and Becky Spore corroborated Colleen's testimony. Pat's mother told of Mike having lunch at home most work days so as to be with his wife, how Pat always kept the two little girls so well dressed and with every hair in place that "I used to think, gee, Pat and the kids can just go to the photographers and have their portrait taken." She told of Pat's purchase of Rely on a shopping trip and of Pat's illness and in receiving a call that "we lost our baby."

Pat's best friend, Becky, told the jury how excited Pat was about the Amway program, how happy she had looked the Wednesday before she died. P&G did not cross-examine Mrs. Robinson. The only question asked of Becky was whether Pat had mentioned working outside the house other than as an Amway dealer. Becky said Pat had not.

Pathologist Francis Skopec, M.D., stated Jacobs told him he believed he had a TSS case when he requested the autopsy. The autopsy showed Pat was having her period and that a layer of bacteria could be seen in the cervix. The IUD had three kinds of bacteria on it, *Staph aureus*, *E coli* and *Strep D*. It was Skopec's opinion that the IUD picked up the bacteria when it was removed by way of the vagina. The uterus seemed free of bacterial infection. The pathologist expressed his belief that tampons play a role in TSS when *Staph aureus* is present.

On cross-examination, Skopec admitted that the diagnosis of TSS was based on Jacobs's diagnosis and not on the autopsy.

On redirect examination, he readily agreed his autopsy findings were consistent with TSS.

Dr. Earl E. Haas, inventor of Tampax, had died five months after I had taken his deposition. I asked Max Hahn to read Haas's answers to the deposition questions. Hahn was a local celebrity. For years he had hosted a children's television show, and he was still active in the community theater. Hahn found the Haas role to be irresistible and his inflections of Haas's answers, as well as the answers themselves, gave the jury some comic relief after the emotionally wrenching testimony of Pat Kehm's sister, mother and best friend.

Haas had said he coined the name Tampax by combining the words tampon and pack because "when a woman patient had a lot of bleeding after delivery, we would tampon her or pack her, with cotton." Jurors smiled when they heard Haas's account of how he had sold his invention of Tampax for $32,000 in 1936, retaining no royalties on what became a billion dollar industry. Since Rely was designed to occlude or block off the menstrual flow, Haas's statement that his cotton Tampax was designed to absorb, not block the flow, as nature intended, was key to our argument.

As the first week of trial ended, I called an economist who testified as to the economic value of a housewife and mother. The witness calculated that the annual value of Pat Kehm's services in 1980 was $12,600. Projected into the future, the economic loss to Mike Kehm and the two children as a result of Pat's premature death was $765,000 according to the economist. He took future inflation into account in making the projection. He also testified that his valuation of loss was a purely economic one and did not include the loss of noneconomic services such as companionship, moral support, love and affection.

On cross-examination, the witness admitted that he had been consulted on approximately two hundred lawsuits, mostly for plaintiffs. He also conceded that he had arrived at the value of $765,000 based upon the cost of replacement for the services regardless of whether Mike actually paid for the replacement. P&G hoped that the jury would pick up on the fact that there would be no need for replacement cost to Mike if he remarried. The P&G attorney questioned the economist's inclusion of the value of chauffeur and maid services:

> "I don't see a lot of limousines driving up and down our streets, so I just wondered if maybe you had—?"
>
> "Well, there again, you are making an assumption that a chauffeur must drive a limousine, but aside from that, I don't see many either."

P&G argued that $100,000 would earn $13,000 per year, which could pay for the $12,600 value of services.

The economist pointed out that P&G could not predict the interest on $100,000 earning $13,000 because inflation and interest rates were not static.

The trial was entering its second week when I called Dr. Gerald Shirk to the stand. Pat's obstetrician-gynecologist had seen her on August 27, 1980, for a pelvic exam following his placement of an IUD on July 15, 1980. He told the jury Pat had been in excellent health ten days before her death. In his opinion, the tampon, not the IUD, was responsible for her death. Shirk also refuted P&G's contention that Jacobs had come up with a diagnosis of TSS after our telephone conversation. Shirk said that Jacobs had told him the day after Pat Kehm died that he felt she had TSS.

On cross-examination, Shirk admitted that TSS occurred in males and nonmenstruating women.

Noting that the pathologist found infection and erosion of the cervix, Woodside asked:

"And isn't it true, sir, that one of the adverse reactions associated with the Copper 7 intrauterine device is erosion or infection of the cervix?"

"Correct."

Woodside concluded his cross-examination on a high point by having Shirk read from the CDC's *MMWR* of September 19, 1980:

"Although the use of tampons is undoubtedly an important factor in the development of TSS in menstruating women, the pathogenesis of TSS is not yet fully understood."

"What does the word pathogenesis mean, sir?" Woodside asked.

"That means the complete reason why women develop Toxic Shock Syndrome," the doctor answered.

"And that wasn't known on September 19th, 1980, was it, sir?"

"No."

"And as a matter of fact, it's not known, today?"

"Correct," Shirk acknowledged.

After Shirk stepped down, I called my last witness. More than a year and a half had passed since his wife's death. Mike Kehm was finally having his day in court. With occasional glances to his right where the jury sat, Mike traced his life as a child growing up in Cedar Rapids, his learning the automotive mechanics trade and then his life with Pat Kehm, whom he met in January 1973, when she was still a high school senior. Smiling nervously, he told how they had begun steady dating and how he gave Pat a diamond engagement ring for Christmas 1973. He described the close relationship he had developed with Pat's mother and her sister Colleen even before the young couple married in November 1974. He spoke of their love, which they extended to their children. I asked:

"What did Pat do to make your life and your children's life more comfortable?"

"Pat was a giver, not a taker. She always put us first. She always had the meals ready on time. The normal domestic type chores, laundry, those types of things."

"When you came home from work, what did you find?"

"I can't hardly ever recall her not having the evening meal ready, of course, herself presentable. I have never walked in and seen her in a bathrobe or curlers. The house was always in good order."

He told of how he and Pat became Amway distributors so Pat's dream house would become attainable earlier, about the Labor Day weekend, their last weekend together, when they took the children to a park. He described Pat's illness from its onset until they went to the Mercy emergency room around midnight on September 5, 1980.

"Twice while we were there that evening she vomited. She was miserable. I know she wasn't comfortable at all laying on that hard examining couch in the emergency room."

"Had you ever seen her that ill before in your life?"

"Not as long as I had known Pat, no. I had never seen her like that."

With obvious anguish, he described the next day with Pat, as sick as she was, bathing in order to be presentable. He told how they had trouble getting even a loose pair of his old blue jeans on her—she had not wanted to wear shorts because she was self-conscious about her discolored legs. He told the jury he had never heard of TSS or problems with tampons. As far as he knew, Pat hadn't heard of it either.

Mike then recounted the hours at the hospital, when he alternated between holding his wife's hands and pacing the waiting room floor. He recalled a discussion with Jacobs about tampons and the disease he had never heard of before that day—Toxic Shock Syndrome. He told how the family priest was not allowed to see Pat because the doctor thought it might scare her if she thought the last rites were to be administered, and he described Pat's worsening condition and then her death.

"Were those confusing times for you?"

"Yeah. There was times I know for the next week or two that certain things didn't register on me until two or three days later. I was—you know, it was a week after Pat had died before I realized who had the girls during those times. It just—I was in a state of confusion."

"Where were you staying at the time?"

"With my parents. I stayed there—I never went back to our home."

"At least not to live, you mean?"

"Not to live, that's correct."

In addition to finding the Rely box he had thrown in the wastebasket, he told of a single Rely tampon he found in Pat's purse while cleaning out a closet at their Bowling Street home. He recalled a discussion with Pat a short time before her death.

"It was rather ironic that several weeks before Pat's death we somehow got on the morbid subject of what would happen to one of us, what we wanted the other person to do and so on, and we weren't even really being half serious at the time, but she mentioned that 'Don't ever split the girls up. If you need help, have Colleen help you.'"

"After Pat's death, did Colleen offer to help out?"

"That was one of the first things she said to me when she found out that Pat had died, that she would do everything she could to help me with the girls."

He was asked why he had filed a claim for punitive damages, which he had added to his lawsuit in December of 1980.

"Because they let my wife die, and, as I understand it, punitive damages are to punish."

Mike told the jury he added the punitive damages claim after finding out that P&G had been told about the tampon

connection over two months before Pat's illness. I then asked
him about the P&G memo of June 27, 1980, to their salesmen,
which described the symptoms of TSS as fever of 102 degrees
or higher, vomiting and diarrhea, rash and low blood pressure.
Mike testified that his wife had had all of those symptoms.

I then asked him about the memo:

> "And then after they described all of that (those symp-
> toms), what did they tell their area representatives?"

Mike read the instruction, one that P&G would repeat to
their sales force throughout the summer of 1980:

> "You should not initiate discussion of this subject."

I handed Mike two more P&G memos, the first dated August 6, 1980, exactly one month before Pat Kehm's death.
Mike read:

> "In a discussion I recognize that the likelihood of TSS
> blowing up into a major consumer issue is relatively slim.
> However, are we certain we ought to be committing the
> financial resources to the stockpiling of Rely K prior to
> our having a final point of view from the CDC and the
> FDA on TSS?"

Mike then read the second memo.

> "If a clear correlation between tampon usage and TSS is
> established, and if the mortality rate on TSS increases,
> the tampon business could be in real trouble."

I interrupted:

> "I have shown you many memorandums, have I not, from
> Procter & Gamble Company?"
> "Yes."
> "Have you seen any memorandum that expresses any
> concern about how people would be in trouble if toxic
> shock continued?"

P&G attorneys objected that the question was argumentative, and McManus agreed. Mike then read the last paragraph of the P&G memo:

> "I don't think we should put Rely in neutral for the next year or two—we have momentum behind the brand now which we will never have again. This argues that we should continue our planned activity to support this brand and build its share of leadership status."

Mike read the pertinent part of another P&G memo, this one dated August 8, 1980.

> "Today, we have had bad news. Public relations learned through a reporter from the Worcester, Massachusetts *Evening Gazette* that a woman in that community has died . . . reportedly suffering from TSS. The reporter says the product used was Rely. He seemed to be a responsible reporter and was quite knowledgeable about TSS. He had talked to CDC.
>
> "We are preparing revised responses to press inquiries in the event the Worcester case stirs up more publicity."

I asked Mike to read what P&G claimed, in a memo dated August 20, 1980, its knowledge was about severe illness resulting from Rely tampons.

> "Rely was introduced in 1974, and in all of our extensive pre-market testing and market experience, we have never been aware of any severe illness caused by the use of our product."

I pointed out that the new position paper was written after the memorandum about the Rely death in Massachusetts. It was also written five days after P&G's most recent visit to the CDC. I directed Mike to read what P&G had been told by the CDC on August 15, 1980.

> "Tampon use continues to be strongly associated with the disease in women. While a specific mechanism of action

remains to be demonstrated, the CDC investigators appear to be convinced that the use of tampons promotes and may even be necessary for the disease in those menstruating women who carry organisms and are susceptible."

I handed Mike another P&G memo, this one dated August 18, 1980, and dealing with P&G's decision to continue marketing Rely.

"And what's the answer or decision they reached three weeks before your wife died?" I asked.

Mike read P&G's decision to continue normal promotion:

"If we don't, we can expect Rely's share to decline from its current 15–20% to 5–10%. It would be financially unattractive for Rely to stay in business at this low share level."

Finally, I asked Mike to read what P&G said, three weeks before Pat's death, about its decision not to warn of TSS. The young man read:

"On advertising: As a public service, we could communicate the symptoms of Toxic Shock Syndrome so that women would know they should go to the hospital quickly if they have these symptoms. This option should be considered but is probably premature to do this at this time."

I then asked, "Was it premature for your wife?"
"No."

The P&G attorney, in cross-examining Mike, suggested that his wife might have had some leftover Playtex when her menstrual period started. Mike replied that he "might believe that but for the fact that Friday I stayed home with her and emptied the trash that had accumulated all week and I found no boxes of Playtex in the trash." When pressed further, Mike conceded that he couldn't say that his wife had not used Playtex for the first part of her period.

Hoping to show that Mike would not have discarded the evidence if he felt the tampons were responsible for his wife's illness, the P&G attorney asked:

> "So what did you do with this box and these tampons?"
>
> "In a fit of anger and disgust, she had only been dead maybe an hour and a half, two hours at the most, I picked them up and threw them in the wastebasket which is under the bathroom sink."

Mike had originally sued for $5 million in compensatory damages. When I discovered that P&G knew of the tampon association with TSS, I had added a claim for $25 million for punitive damages. Since a punitive damages award can be based upon the wealth and income of the defendant, McManus had ruled that evidence of P&G's net worth of $5 billion and its after tax income of $643 million the year of Pat's death was admissible in the event the jury decided to award punitive damages. Shortly before the trial, I had struck claims for specific amounts and asked for whatever amount the jury would find proper under the law. I suspected that conservative jurors might be offended by such a large request for damages, no matter how justified it might be under the law. Mike was asked by the P&G attorney:

> "How did you arrive at the $5 million compensatory damages?"
>
> "The figures actually are irrelevant in my mind as far as what I have lost or what—the fact my children will not know their mother's natural love," Mike answered.
>
> "Now, have you ever considered what you might do if this jury gave you $30 million dollars?"
>
> "It's inconceivable in my mind, that large amount of money, sir. I can't answer that. That would be pure speculation."
>
> "Well, have you ever told anybody such as your sister-in-law, Colleen Jones, that you might quit your job at McGrath's?"

"I think I told her that at some point it certainly wasn't going to be necessary for me to have to work ten or ten and a half hours a day any more. I don't believe I told anyone I was going to quit my job."

On redirect examination, I asked Mike about his understanding of punitive damages:

"And what was your understanding, on the basis of what I explained to you, the reason for the punitive damage claim was?"

"I can't talk like a lawyer, but as best as you explained it to me, punitive damages are to punish the defendants so that they won't be tempted to do this again, and my feelings for even having punitive damages is that my wife is dead, but maybe somebody else's life someday could be saved."

With that, I rested my case, and it was now P&G's turn to present its case to the jury.

15

*"We reported to the Board of Directors
what we knew as the information [about
TSS] unfolded in the marketplace . . . by
that I mean around the country . . ."*

P&G Chairman of the Board
Edward Harness, on cross-examination

On Tuesday, April 13, 1982, the seventh day of the trial,
P&G called its first witness—Charles Fullgraf, former company group vice president. Fullgraf had begun his career at
P&G forty-two years earlier, upon graduation from Washington University in St. Louis with a bachelor's degree in chemical engineering. At the time of the trial, his 24,687 shares of
common stock in P&G were worth in excess of $2 million.

Now retired, Fullgraf sat at the counsel table as the representative of P&G and smiled benevolently throughout the trial.
He and general counsel Powell McHenry were the only
P&G representatives to express their condolences to Mike Kehm
for the loss of his wife, but they did so off the stand at the trial
and outside the presence of the jury.

On direct testimony, Fullgraf claimed that P&G "completed exhaustive safety testing on [Rely] and finally took the

tampon into the test market". Calder asked Fullgraf to comment further on testing.

> "At the time Rely was being prepared for market introduction, did Procter & Gamble have a company policy regarding product safety?"
>
> "Yes, we certainly did. That policy has the highest priority, that every product we sell must be safe for the consumer to use."

Calder asked why P&G had taken Rely off the market on September 22, 1980. The veteran P&G executive began his answer:

> "Even though there was not one shred of evidence that Rely—"

Then he caught himself and started over:

> "There was not one shred of scientific evidence that Rely was involved in Toxic Shock Syndrome. We concluded we could not risk the ongoing very bad publicity, and we therefore concluded we should withdraw our product from the market."

During cross-examination, Fullgraf admitted sitting with other P&G executives in Cincinnati headquarters during the summer of 1980 and watching videotape copies of newscasts about TSS cases occurring on the West Coast. But he justified P&G's failure to warn on the basis that P&G did not know how to do so "given the fragmentary information we had."

> "We had no scientific evidence, confirmed scientific evidence, that linked tampons or Rely with Toxic Shock Syndrome," Fullgraf asserted.
>
> "How many women would have had to die before you got scientific evidence to satisfy you and the other corporate officers?" I countered.
>
> MR. CALDER: "Objection."
>
> THE COURT: "What grounds?"

Mr. Calder: "Well, I think it's argumentative for one thing."

The Court: "Sustained."

I felt it was important to show that P&G had done little or nothing to investigate TSS in the summer of 1980. Fullgraf admitted that although he had read Todd's *Lancet* article on TSS in May, P&G did not contact Todd for his views until August 27, 1980, some two months after the CDC I study had been released.

> "Can you tell me what you did in July of 1980, while women were getting sick in America and some were dying with Toxic Shock Syndrome, what did Procter & Gamble do about this problem?"
>
> "We went back and researched the literature as intensely as we knew how."
>
> "That would take about an hour or two, wouldn't it, because there were only two articles written then, Mr. Fullgraf?"

Fullgraf acknowledged that to be the case but claimed it took a long time to establish that fact.

Referring to P&G's "Special Projects Committee," I asked Fullgraf:

> "In his deposition Widder several times referred to it as a Special Problems Committee, which is an understandable mistake, because it was a problem, wasn't it?"
>
> "Yes, sir, and this is a very serious problem."
>
> "Yes. You have lost a product that was successful?"
>
> "Yes, sir."
>
> "And my client has lost his wife?"
>
> "Yes, sir."

Then I brought up P&G's claim during the summer of 1980 that tampons have been around for forty years and they haven't caused any problems:

"And in reliance on that you said tampons have been around for forty years and they haven't caused any problems. That was one of the statements that PR people at Procter & Gamble put out, isn't that right?"

"I believe that was a statement of fact, yes, sir."

"But those weren't the same tampons for the first forty years, were they, Mr. Fullgraf?"

"Not totally, no, sir."

While Fullgraf stubbornly continued to maintain that there was insufficient evidence of a tampon and TSS connection, he was led into a damaging admission:

"If you had a young friend, like a granddaughter or a niece or somebody, who was using tampons in their menstrual period and they developed a fever and some nausea and diarrhea, what would you tell them to do, Mr. Fullgraf?"

"I would tell them to get to their doctor as promptly as they could."

"Wouldn't you tell them something before that?"

"Yes, I would tell them that if they were using a tampon to remove it."

"Did you tell the people that bought your product in the summer of 1980 that?"

"No, sir, we did not."

Fullgraf's cross-examination concluded with the admission that it would have cost somewhere in the range of a penny or two to put a sticker on a Rely package warning about TSS.

P&G's next witness was Dr. Tommy Evans, from the Department of Obstetrics and Gynecology at Wayne State University in Detroit. Evans's testimony was supposed to create the impression in the jurors' minds that little was known about TSS even in 1982—thereby letting P&G off the hook for its failure to be knowledgeable about TSS in the summer of 1980.

Recognizing that Evans might be sensitive about his longstanding relationship with P&G, I first asked him about his financial arrangements with the company. Then, hoping that Evans's self-esteem and sense of integrity were more important than the money he received, I asked him:

> "Doctor, you want to retain your objectivity despite the fact that you are funded from time to time by Procter & Gamble, isn't that right?"
>
> "Yes, I hold my reputation to honesty, and it's very important to me."
>
> "And it's also important for you to testify as to the best of your judgment and ability at this time?"
>
> "That's correct."
>
> "Don't you believe in connection with this objectivity that tampons play some kind of a role as a co-factor or otherwise in Toxic Shock Syndrome in menstruating women?"
>
> "It certainly appears to be so."

I could now argue in summation to the jury that if a P&G expert thinks circumstantial evidence points to tampon involvement with TSS, how could a jury find it otherwise?

After Evans left the stand, P&G called Gordon Hassing, a Ph.D. in biochemistry from the University of Michigan. But a few minutes after he began his testimony, it was interrupted by the arrival of Dr. James Todd. Hassing stepped down so the discoverer of TSS could give his testimony without waiting.

Under direct examination by Woodside, Todd acknowledged being the doctor who first defined the entity Toxic Shock Syndrome in the article published in *Lancet* in 1978. He told how he had received a grant from P&G to do research, which paid $403,000 over a two-year period. He charged P&G $400 per hour for testifying in court, including travel time, but said that the money goes to the Denver Children's Hospital.

Todd told how Dr. Kathryn Shands of the CDC contacted him in February 1980 after receiving reports from health departments in Minnesota, Wisconsin, Illinois and Utah of cases that looked and sounded like TSS. She came to see Todd in

Denver, and they worked out a tentative case definition of TSS, which evolved into the CDC case definition. Woodside went through a litany of questions eliciting the answer that TSS has been found in individuals who are not menstruating, in males, in menstruating women who use sanitary napkins or mini-pads, in menstruating women who use sea sponges, in postpartum women, in both male and female post operative patients, in women who have had IUDs, in women using diaphragms, in women who have had breast implants, in patients with boils and abscesses, in patients with nasal infections and in cases of husbands and wives simultaneously. Todd agreed with Woodside that it has not been scientifically established that tampons cause TSS.

Woodside asked Todd about a P&G memo that I had previously introduced into evidence—one that showed that Todd had told P&G on August 27, 1980, that he believed that tampons are a cofactor because they operate as a "functional abscess." Woodside then asked:

> "Dr. Todd, has it been scientifically shown, to the best of your knowledge, that a tampon functions as a functional abscess?"
> "No."

Todd testified that he was critical of the CDC II study. It was presented in a fragmentary form in the *MMWR*, he asserted. It was difficult for him to evaluate those results because the CDC presented its results and conclusions but said little about its methods. Also, he felt there were a number of potential biases in the study.

Satisfied with that answer, Woodside turned Todd over for cross-examination.

I got Todd to admit that after receiving the $403,000 grant from P&G, he had written an editorial in *Pediatrics* magazine using the term "toxic schlock." Todd agreed that the $403,000 was the largest grant he had ever received from a business firm for research. Though he was grateful to P&G, he admitted he was concerned about being marked as a P&G man and that that had actually happened.

Referring to Woodside's direct examination about IUDs, I asked:

> "Now, with respect to IUD's, you do not believe that IUD's cause Toxic Shock Syndrome, do you?"
> "No."

Intending to end my cross-examination on a high point, I asked:

> "And, Doctor, as one of the most knowledgeable people on Toxic Shock Syndrome, as you sit here today, you believe that tampons play a role in causing Toxic Shock Syndrome in menstruating women, don't you?"
> "I believe that they are involved in the pathogenesis of the disease in some patients with Toxic Shock Syndrome."

When Hassing returned to the stand following the conclusion of Todd's testimony, he dropped an unexpected bombshell. I couldn't believe my ears.

Calder had asked Hassing if Bruce Dan or anyone else with the CDC ever suggested that P&G should adopt some type of TSS warning. I expected Hassing to say that the CDC had not directed P&G or the other tampon companies to put warning labels on their boxes. I wouldn't have been surprised at such an answer because it wasn't in CDC's authority to regulate the tampon companies. That responsibility belonged to the FDA. However, I was not prepared for the claim Hassing was about to make.

In response to Calder's question about whether the CDC suggested a warning be given, Hassing boldly replied:

> "No, they did not. It was quite to the contrary. I distinctly remember a meeting I was at on August 21 at CDC. It involved Dr. Shands and Dr. Dan and Dr. Schmid, and I was struck by the fact that after we had

discussed other aspects of Toxic Shock Syndrome, that Dr. Shands, who was a very young women herself, indicated very strongly that she was not going to change her tampon habits, and she was going to keep using tampons, and she specifically didn't see the need for a warning."

I was stunned by Hassing's testimony. Our punitive damages claim now lay in shreds. The crux of it had rested on the premise that P&G showed a reckless and wanton disregard for human life when it failed in the summer of 1980 to warn Rely users about the risk of TSS. With Shands, the government's top expert on TSS, telling P&G as late as August 21, 1980, that a warning was not necessary, how could it reasonably be argued that P&G's failure to warn rose to the level of a wanton disregard for human life? P&G might still be liable for compensatory damages for having a defective product but not punitive damages. I felt Hassing was probably lying—he hadn't mentioned the conversation when I took his deposition the previous summer. But I told Mike there was nothing we could do about it—and Hassing knew it—because of the government policy against permitting CDC personnel to testify in civil cases while they were still employed with the CDC. We couldn't call Shands to rebut whatever Hassing attributed to her—a golden opportunity for Hassing to say whatever helped P&G win the case.

After court was over that day, I called Bruce Dan and asked if he remembered any conversation like the one Hassing had described. Dan said it was quite likely that Shands had told Hassing she would still continue to use tampons because of their convenience coupled with the fact she knew how to recognize the incipient signs of TSS and what to do if they appeared. However, he couldn't imagine Shands telling any tampon company not to warn about TSS. He explained that that would be contrary to what the CDC task force on TSS had been trying to do in educating the public about TSS during the summer of 1980. He promised to double-check with

Shands to satisfy my curiosity even though Shands would not be available to testify. Dan called back to say that he had talked with Shands, and she denied ever saying anything remotely resembling the warning statement, although, as Dan predicted, she saw no reason to stop using tampons and may well have told Hassing that. Dan asked if he could testify as to what Shands told him, and I advised that the hearsay rule would not allow his testimony on that point. We agreed it was a travesty of justice that would allow Hassing's claim to go unchallenged, but our hands seemed to be tied.

The next morning, I told Mike there was nothing we could do about the harm done to the punitive damages claim, and that I hoped it wouldn't spill over onto our compensatory damages claim as well.

During his direct examination, Hassing also spoke of various meetings with the FDA up until and after Rely was withdrawn from the marketplace. The day after the withdrawal, September 23, 1980, P&G met again with the FDA. Hassing said that P&G told the FDA that the company was going to study TSS very carefully:

> "We were upset that so little was known, and we were going to establish a scientific program where we would support scientists with independent grants . . . we would pledge several million dollars to do that, and in fact that's what we did."

What I didn't know during the trial and what I presume the FDA still doesn't know was that the funding was part of its defense of TSS litigation and that checks for grants were issued through the P&G legal defense fund checking account.

Hassing claimed that the funding was humanitarian and that the money would be "unrestricted." All P&G asked, he said, was that "we would have an opportunity to visit them periodically, to learn about what they were actually doing, and we would want to see copies of any manuscripts that they would prepare for the scientific literature twenty-one days before they would mail it off, just so that we would know what the contents of the paper would be."

Calder ended his examination of Hassing by asking him about cases of TSS in foreign countries. Hassing stated that Canada has a large number of cases, and Calder asked him:

> "Has Rely ever been sold in Sweden?"
> "Rely has never been sold outside the United States."

I questioned Hassing about the FDA, whom Hassing earlier had cited as being supportive of the P&G testing and marketing of Rely. Intending to show that the FDA was less than diligent in protecting consumer interests where tampons are concerned, I asked if it was true that the FDA, as of the trial in April 1982, still had not required warnings. Hassing claimed the FDA was supposed to make a final ruling on the subject soon.

> "Not exactly setting any records for moving along, are they?" I asked.
> "Well, it is their business. I don't know what their record is."
> "Canada, on the other hand, they adopted a requirement in 1980, didn't they?"
> "They adopted a requirement. I can't tell you when they did it."

Under cross-examination, Hassing admitted that Rely did not have to have FDA approval under the Medical Devices Act because it had been "grandfathered in"; it had been sold in the marketplace prior to passage of the act in May of 1976. In the summer of 1980, the FDA was bombarded with an organized letter campaign to require ingredient labeling on tampons. When Yin contacted P&G about this in August, Hassing took the position that it was "not useful to the consumer" to have ingredient labeling. I asked Hassing:

"What possible harm can come from your company putting the ingredients on a package of a product that is in-
serted into an orifice of the body?"

"We told Dr. Yin that we would—"

"Excuse me," I interrupted Hassing. "I would like a
direct answer. I am asking you a question."

Turning to the court, I said:

"I would like to ask the witness to answer."

> HASSING: "I would like to answer the question with
> what we actually told Dr. Yin."
>
> "I would like to know what the harm is. I don't care
> what you told Dr. Yin," I persisted.
>
> THE COURT: "You can tell later what you told Dr.
> Yin."

Hassing still avoided my question by answering:

> "We did give that information to consumers when they
> called or wrote."

I drew from Hassing the admission that while P&G had
not informed the public about the tampon association with
TSS, they had informed their sales representatives about it in
June of 1980 when they instructed them not to initiate the
subject with doctors:

> "It is kind of interesting when you think about it. Your
> sales representatives, if one of their family members had
> gotten a fever and nausea and diarrhea while they were
> using a tampon, would recognize that they might have
> Toxic Shock Syndrome, wouldn't they, as a result of being
> informed by a memorandum dated June 27, 1980?"
>
> "They would know it," Hassing admitted, "but the
> public would have known it from reports in the press,"
> he argued.

But I reminded him that a P&G study in August 1980 found that only 20 percent of American women had even heard about TSS.

Hassing admitted that during the summer of 1980, Rely continued to increase its share in the tampon market because P&G was advertising it extensively over radio, television and in the newspapers and magazines and that in July P&G sent out two and a half million free samples of Rely. Hassing also admitted that women participating in a Rely clinical study in late summer of 1980 were not told of the possible TSS danger until after the publicity came out surrounding CDC II.

I told Hassing I had seen P&G memos from the summer of 1980 expressing concern about what would happen to the tampon industry if TSS continued. I asked Hassing if there were any memos issued that summer that expressed any concern about what might be happening to the health of American women. Hassing answered that he didn't know about a specific memorandum to that effect.

Remembering Hassing's statement that there were TSS cases in Canada and that the product had not been sold there, I asked if P&G had cooperated with the FDA in the summer and fall of 1980 and Hassing answered yes. I asked, at that time, had Hassing ever misrepresented facts or given false information to the FDA? Hassing answered that he had not. I then showed Hassing a letter that he had written to the FDA on September 23, 1980. The letter stated that TSS had occurred in areas where Rely was not marketed, such as Canada, and that P&G did not market Rely outside the United States. I also reminded Hassing that he had made a similar representation to the jury on direct examination.

I then handed him an exhibit that was a memorandum to Hassing, dated September 22, 1980, the day before Hassing's letter to the FDA. I asked Hassing to read the memo that contained the statement that the Canadian Health Protection Branch knew about the second CDC Study and had received a report about a sixteen-year-old girl having TSS symptoms three times while using Rely. The memo went on:

"We expect to be able to get Rely off retail shelves in Canada within a few days."

Turning my back on Hassing's flushed face, I told the court that that concluded my cross-examination.

Upon redirect examination by Calder, Hassing said that P&G did not sell Rely in Canada but that he was aware that there was wholesale purchasing in the United States by third parties for resale in Canada. Regarding the sale of Rely without carboxymethylcellulose (CMC) in Japan, Hassing claimed that Japan had a "rather obscure performance standard, that included a test in which a tampon would be put in water and the investigator would look for material that would fall off such as pieces of cotton or rayon that might remain behind in the woman's vagina." The way Japan did the test, Hassing explained, they measured the amount of residue that was left after the water was evaporated rather than measuring the amount of material that physically fell off. He conceded that enough solubles came out of the CMC in Rely that at times it would pass the test and at other times it would fail. Hassing concluded by suggesting that P&G decided to remove CMC from the products sold in Japan "rather than try and change the standard with the government of Japan or try to get a better interpretation of the standard because even without carboxymethylcellulose the Rely product would be superior to any product that was in Japan at that time."

At the noon recess, I showed Mike Kehm a letter that had been written by the director of the Bacterial Diseases Division of the CDC to the Health Industry Manufacturers Association. The letter sought financial funding from the tampon trade group to answer remaining questions about tampons and TSS. P&G was contending that the letter should be admitted as rebuttal to Dan and Tierno. I argued that it did not rebut Dan and Tierno because neither expert said that all the questions about tampons and TSS had been answered. By ruling in our favor, the court agreed that it wasn't proper rebuttal and, further, that it had not been on the pretrial exhibit list.

The letter stated that because of financial limitations the CDC would not achieve all of its objectives as rapidly as it might wish. It solicited money from the tampon companies' trade association to conduct further research and indicated that the CDC would be pleased to send reports concerning the results of such research to the association. Mike and I reflected on the shame and irony that it was necessary for our government to have to beg for funds for research from the very parties that created the health problem. As we read the letter, however, we noted that, to the CDC's credit, it concluded: "There will, however, be no control over how the gift will be allocated to achieve the stated objectives." P&G and the other tampon companies were not interested—not on those terms.

The Yale expert in epidemiology, Alvan R. Feinstein, demonstrated his courtroom experience or his prepping by turning toward the jury each time he answered questions. In spite of this practice, and his folksy manner, he may have alienated the jurors by describing the American Epidemiological Society, of which he was a member, as "kind of an elitist group in the field of epidemiology." He told the jury there were a number of different potential biases that, in his opinion, rendered all of the tampon and TSS studies invalid. He lumped the different studies together because they all used the same case-control method. In Feinstein's judgment, there were possible biases or errors in diagnoses by the physician, the victim's uncertainty about tampon brand use and the prejudice of the person asking the questions of the cases and controls.

He cited *Lancet* articles that found a substantial risk for breast cancer in women using Reserpine, a drug for treating high blood pressure. He said that studies done in the United States, England and Finland all showed the same elevated risk, following which there was a "large outcry" to have Reserpine removed from the market because of its possible role as a carcinogen. Feinstein claimed that subsequent studies tended to exonerate Reserpine, and it became apparent that the original studies, examined more closely, contained various built-in distortions. Feinstein felt that the same criticisms could be made about the CDC Studies and the others from the State Health Department. He was asked:

> "Do you know what lies behind the numbers in the Toxic Shock Syndrome studies?"
>
> "All I can say is that in terms of the usual scientific precautions that I would have expected or have wanted to see, those precautions weren't used," Feinstein answered.

On cross-examination, I asked if Feinstein had contacted Bruce Dan for any information about how the CDC carried out its studies. He had not. His information was secondhand. Even when he talked with Osterholm, the head of the Tri-State Study, Feinstein admitted that he had personally not discussed the methods of that study.

Feinstein admitted that case-control studies can be an important research tool in the study of disease, and that he did not fault the CDC in June of 1980 for conducting a case-control retrospective study. I also gained the concession that since people were getting very sick and in some cases dying, a retrospective case study made more sense in connection with TSS than a prospective study. He conceded that if a study has been well done, fifty cases are enough to make it valid.

One of Feinstein's criticisms of CDC I was that it had not published the total number of TSS cases CDC started with before they picked the fifty for the study. My legal assistant, Michele, called my attention to an article about the CDC I findings from the *New England Journal of Medicine*. I handed the article to the witness and asked him to read a certain passage. What Feinstein had supposedly searched for—the number of TSS cases that CDC started out with and the number that was excluded when the CDC I Study was carried out—was right there in front of him.

To counter Feinstein's claim that massive publicity about TSS distorted CDC II, I showed him a late July P&G memo that revealed only 5 percent of American women had heard of a tampon connection with Toxic Shock Syndrome. I asked

Feinstein to read to the jury how many of the respondents named any particular tampon brand in connection with medical problems. Feinstein read:

> "Very few of these respondents named any particular brand in connection with medical problems and none of them named Rely."

When Feinstein countered that massive publicity wasn't affecting women particularly but that it was affecting physicians, I showed him a P&G study of September 1980 indicating that physicians were ill-informed about TSS and were not identifying or recognizing the symptoms.

I ended my cross-examination by reminding Feinstein of a sworn statement he had made in an affidavit to help P&G persuade the court to keep out evidence of the CDC studies. He had claimed that a bias could grow out of the fact that TSS victims who were asked to recommend friends as controls "might be more likely to choose a friend who does not use tampons in order to help prove the case against tampons."

> "Isn't that what you said?"
> "That is possible."
> "That is kind of paranoic, isn't it?"
> "Not necessarily."

As I sat down, Mike Kehm said to me: "Everytime they bring somebody on against us, you knock 'em down like a bowling ball." I reminded him that that wasn't true with respect to refuting Hassing's testimony about Shands, yet I thought things had gone pretty well, too. Here was this Eastern elitist, Feinstein, who had not carefully read an important article in the *New England Journal of Medicine*. And then there was his paranoia. Still, I couldn't get Mrs. Beauregard out of my head. She kept smiling every time Woodside did something clever. And the verdict had to be unanimous.

After Feinstein, P&G called microbiologist Widder, chemistry safety expert Owen Carter and the P&G associate director of Product Development, Martin Cannon, to testify. These employees supported the official P&G position that Rely had been carefully tested from a safety standpoint before being sold in the marketplace, that they had no reason to suspect there was anything about tampons in general, and Rely in particular, that would make them unsafe for American women and that, in the case of Cannon and Carter, they still believed that.

Cannon also corroborated Hassing's testimony about Shands saying she saw no reason to warn. Cannon wasn't in Atlanta and, therefore, didn't hear Shands say it. But he testified that Hassing, on his return from the CDC, told Cannon about it.

Although there was the incentive of winning the case for Hassing to fabricate the Shands statement during the Kehm trial, there was no reason for him to do so upon his return from Atlanta in August 1980. Since Shands didn't say it and Hassing would have had no reason at that time to say she did, then where did Cannon get the notion that he did? The most plausible explanation is that Cannon, who admits he read transcripts of witnesses who testified before him, picked up on what Hassing claimed he heard and embellished on it, or he may have heard about it during the secret mock trials in Lincoln, Nebraska. But since I couldn't get Shands as a witness to rebut it, it didn't really matter what inspired Cannon to recall something that would not have been said.

Widder admitted that he said at his deposition that tampons appeared to have a role to play in TSS and menstruating women, but he qualified it at trial. His opinion was based on the epidemiological studies of the CDC and other state public health agencies, which he now felt were questionable in light of Feinstein's analyses for potential biases.

P&G then turned to an Iowa boy who had made good in the field of science—Patrick Schlievert. Schlievert had received a B.A. in geology in 1971 from the University of Iowa. In 1976, he obtained a Ph.D. in microbiology from Iowa. He taught at the University of Minnesota for three years before accepting a position at UCLA as assistant professor of microbiology. At the time he testified in the Kehm case, he was back at the University of Minnesota.

P&G wanted to use Schlievert to attack Tierno's theories about TSS. The two scientists had engaged in a not-so-polite debate on the subject at a meeting of microbiologists in Atlanta, several weeks earlier—and Schlievert was all too eager to come to Iowa and tell the jury what he thought of Tierno. Osterholm had warned me about this.

Unfortunately for P&G, Schlievert had not been on their original expert witness list. Since he had been added as a late witness, the judge decided he would be allowed as a rebuttal witness to Bruce Dan, but not Tierno, because Dan, unlike Tierno, was added to our witness list after the deadline.

Several scientists confided to me that Schlievert enjoyed publicity and that he would make bold statements to the news media and then later deny quotes that came back to haunt him. After the trial, I learned that Schlievert had contacted John Carlson, a reporter, the night before he testified, offering to give an interview. Since he wouldn't be allowed to rebut Tierno's testimony from the witness box, he told Carlson he would do so in the interview. Carlson, a *Des Moines Register* reporter, who was also covering the trial for the *Wall Street Journal*, declined the offer and said he would write his stories on what was said under oath from the witness stand. Before court began the next morning, Woodside inquired of Carlson if he had gotten together with Schlievert. The reporter merely smiled. While on the witness stand, Schlievert would attribute an embarrassing news story quote to the fact that he was usually misquoted by the press—an irony that was lost on me because I didn't know of his abortive effort hours earlier to attack Tierno in the press.

The gist of Schlievert's testimony was that Rely tampons do not cause Toxic Shock Syndrome but that *Staph aureus* does. Schlievert further testified that there was not sufficient scientific knowledge available in the summer and fall of 1980 to require tampon manufacturers to warn tampon users of a possible association between Toxic Shock Syndrome and tampon use. He testified that on August 14, 1980, the CDC had called him to an Atlanta meeting to find out what he knew about TSS. He said he heard no statement at the CDC that tampon manufacturers should warn women who use tampons about the possibility of developing TSS. He said he tested Rely tampons in the presence of *Staph aureus* "and the components didn't significantly increase toxin production."

Schlievert said that all evidence indicates that the TSS toxin producing the strain of *Staph aureus* is a new strain. He also indicated that some women do not have antibodies to the toxin and they are susceptible to getting TSS.

On cross-examination, Schlievert agreed that approximately 15 to 20 percent of the women in America do not have the antibodies. Schlievert admitted that his friend and colleague, Osterholm, stated publicly in the Tri-State Study that there is an increased risk of TSS with tampons. Although there was no scientific proof of a tampon connection with TSS, I pointed out to Schlievert that there was also no scientific proof that *Staph aureus* is the bacterium responsible for TSS but that Schlievert believes it is nonetheless. Concluding my cross-examination, Schlievert admitted that he had completed one P&G grant and was working on another.

P&G's next witness, Herbert Ley, Jr., M.D., had been Commissioner of the Food and Drug Administration in 1968. When his term expired in December 1969, he had not been reappointed, which is customary whenever there is a change in administration. However, Ley suggested to the jury that he was forced out of the position because he was on the Nixon White House enemies' list. Later, a newspaper reporter observed that there hadn't been a White House enemies' list in late 1969.

Ley started up a consulting business for firms having dealings with the FDA. At the time of the trial, his business, Herbert L. Ley Associates, was in its third year as consultant to P&G for its new drug product development effort. He charged P&G $1,000 a day for such work but estimated that, over the past three years, he had billed them only about $7,000. He told the jury that P&G did more than was required by the FDA in conducting clinical studies of Rely. In his opinion, P&G had no obligation to warn of a possible association between tampon use and TSS.

On cross-examination, I pointed out that since the FDA had no minimum regulations for tampons, it would not be difficult to comply. Ley also agreed that P&G did not have to get FDA approval to put a warning label on its product. On the FDA's laxity in requiring a TSS warning, Ley weakly responded that there is only a proposal that has not yet been made into a regulation.

As the trial began its third week, P&G called its next to last witness, chairman of the executive committee of the board of P&G, Edward Harness.

After the second CDC study had come out in September 1980, Harness had the ultimate responsibility for the decision to recall Rely. According to Harness, P&G made the decision because:

> "No matter what the true medical facts may be, the controversy was dangerous to our company, dangerous to the interests of our company . . ."

On cross-examination, I called Harness's attention to the fact that he had not mentioned any concern about the interest of the consumer in the recall decision—only that of the company. Harness disagreed. But he admitted that the uncertainty about TSS and tampons did not cause P&G to slow down promotion. The company spent millions of advertising dollars on Rely during the summer of 1980.

> "By the way, didn't the June MMWR say some recommendations can be made? Women who have Toxic Shock Syndrome should probably not use tampons for several cycles. Didn't they say that?"
> "Yes," the witness replied.
> "You didn't tell your customers that, did you?"
> "We did not," the P&G board chairman conceded.
> "Didn't they also say, 'Because use of tampons contin-

uously through the period is associated with increased risk of toxic shock, women who wish to decrease the small risk of toxic shock may choose to use tampons during only part of the period or use napkins or mini-pads instead.' Weren't those words found in the MMWR?"

"Yes, I believe they were."

"And you did not tell your customers that, did you?"

"We did not," Harness admitted.

Speaking for P&G, Harness said the giant soap company had done nothing wrong.

"It is Procter & Gamble's claim that Rely is safe and Procter & Gamble has done no wrong. Is that right?" I asked.

"That is the way we felt in the summer of 1980, and the way we still feel," Harness contended.

"Mr. Harness, has Procter & Gamble ever admitted fault or apologized to any victim of Toxic Shock Syndrome or the next of kin?"

"Not to my knowledge."

Harness defended P&G's policy to withhold information about TSS unless someone asked.

"That is what you were doing nationally, not telling anybody about Toxic Shock Syndrome when you sold the product, but if they happened to call in and initiated it, then you would give them information. Isn't that the state of the record?"

"If they called or wrote it, yes."

"But if they weren't informed enough to do that, they were just out of luck, weren't they?"

"Conceivably, yes," Harness acknowledged.

I was certain Harness's advertising background was responsible for his next slip of the tongue:

". . . we reported to the Board of Directors what we knew as the information unfolded in the marketplace."

I was amazed by his reference in that context to the market-place. I wondered if I heard him correctly, so I asked:

"Was that 'in the marketplace?'"

To my amazement, he explained:

"Yes. By that, I mean around the country, you know."

"The country is the marketplace?" I asked, still incredulous that he would visualize the world's oldest existing democracy as simply a "marketplace."

"That is right, in the sense I have used the word," he freely acknowledged.

The defense's last witness, P&G's in-house physician Dr. C. Elizabeth McKinivan, would drop a second bombshell on our case. Looking the jury straight in the eye, McKinivan testified that Pat Kehm died of a bacterial infection in her uterus probably associated with the IUD, and not TSS from a tampon. She based her opinion on the contention that the pathologist, Francis Skopec, had found an infection in the uterus.

Despite the contrary opinions of Pat's treating physicians, she stood her ground. She claimed she was in as good a position to make the diagnosis as the doctors who had actually physically seen and treated Pat Kehm, both when she was healthy as well as on the day she died.

McKinivan admitted she had never treated a patient of her own for TSS. Testifying for P&G in the Lampshire case she told the Denver jury that Ms. Lampshire had something other than TSS. She had not examined Ms. Lampshire either. Later, McKinivan's name would appear as a witness in other TSS cases. In case after case defended by P&G, McKinivan would be listed as a witness who would testify that the victim bringing suit had something other than TSS.

McKinivan based her opinion about Pat Kehm on the autopsy report and the hospital records and claimed she had not read the transcripts of the testimony of Jacobs or Quetsch or the pathologist, Skopec, all of whom had testified that there was no infection in the uterus. If McKinivan was to be believed, P&G had wasted the $25,000 it was spending on "dailies."

I had objected to the court allowing McKinivan to give a diagnosis of Pat Kehm's medical condition. P&G had misled us about the scope of her testimony. I pointed to the witness list, which showed that McKinivan would merely testify to the fact that based on her hospital and medical records, Pat Kehm's symptoms were inconsistent with TSS. I argued that it is one thing to say that the hospital records do not support a particular disease, but that it is quite another to say that the records support a different disease. McManus overruled my objection and permitted McKinivan to give her opinion as to the cause of Pat Kehm's death. After McKinivan completed her testimony, P&G rested.

It was now late in the day, and I called Charles Helms, M.D., to the stand. Helms had been listed as a witness by P&G but not called. Over the weekend, I had gone to Iowa City to see if Helms would testify as an expert in rebuttal in the Kehm case. Helms was troubled by P&G's attacks on the epidemiological studies, particularly Feinstein's testimony that the studies were all one and the same. Helms was willing to testify but insisted that he not be compensated in any way for his participation in the Kehm case—which, in itself, would be a novelty for the jury.

Helms had graduated with honors from Rochester Medical School and did his residency at the prestigious Massachusetts General Hospital in Boston. Prior to coming to the University of Iowa College of Medicine, in July 1976, as director of clinical programs for the Department of Internal Medicine, he had worked at the National Institutes of Health.

Helms told the jury that he did not know he had been listed as a P&G witness. He said he became aware of TSS in May 1980, when he treated a woman in the intensive care unit. At the same time, the *MMWR* came out with its first report on TSS. I then asked him to assume that a patient died on September 6, 1980, of TSS, was examined the night before in the emergency room and no rash was observed or noted by the emergency room physician, would this be unusual or extraordinary?

"It would not be unusual in my experience, no," Helms said.

"Tell the jury why that is," I asked.

"The rash of Toxic Shock Syndrome can be missed for several reasons. One is the geographic location of the rash. It tends to be in the area of the perineum initially, and also in the area of the chest, so that if a doctor doesn't undress the patient, it can be missed."

Helms also testified that another reason it could be missed is the function of tans—a person who has been out in the sun and who is tan will not show the rash very well, he explained. In addition, he said, patients who are in shock have poor profusion, particularly patients who are very ill. The skin will not show this rash very well. He knew of two instances in his experience where the rash had been missed.

I asked Helms what role he had played in the Tri-State Study. He had examined the clinical records of the Iowa cases. At this point, Woodside asked if the lawyers could approach the bench.

A lengthy discussion followed with P&G claiming that the Tri-State Study had been brought up as part of the plaintiff's case and was not a proper subject for rebuttal. I argued it was rebuttal to Feinstein who said that all of the TSS studies were but one study. McManus observed that it was 5:30 p.m., one hour past the usual court adjournment time. I was five minutes from concluding. I told McManus that Helms's rigid schedule would prevent his coming back to court. McManus finally stated he would allow me to ask Helms the one question of whether the Tri-State was a different study from other public health studies. Woodside offered to stipulate that it was more than one study. I responded by asking if P&G would stipulate that Feinstein was wrong. Woodside smiled in response. After more wrangling, McManus decided to allow me to ask Helms about the Tri-State Study.

Helms then testified that the Tri-State was carried out differently from the other studies and that in his opinion it was a valid study and regarded as such by epidemiologists. Woodside interrupted when I asked if Helms could tell the jury in one or two sentences what the Tri-State Study concluded.

> "Your Honor, I believe Mr. Riley was given permission to ask whether it was a separate study."

McManus had forgotten that I'd just asked that question for he responded:

> "Yes, we have had the results of the Tri-State Study, ask him the question."

I then asked Helms about the subject of an article he had recently published in the *American Journal of the Medical Sciences.* Woodside objected and the court sustained the objection. I asked if Helms had made a study of TSS in Iowa and Helms said that he had. I asked Helms to tell the jury as succinctly as he could what that study consisted of. Woodside objected, and the court again sustained the objection. I then asked if the case of Pat Kehm was in that study. Woodside objected, and I responded that the purpose of the question was because the court and jury had just heard testimony from Dr. McKinivan about the diagnosis of Patricia Kehm. The court allowed Helms to answer that Pat Kehm's case was included. When I asked Helms how many cases were in that study, Woodside again approached the bench. I argued that Helms was going to testify that he examined Pat Kehm's records:

> "As a rebuttal to Dr. McKinivan, who comes in with a devastating answer which wasn't in the answers to interrogatories or pretrial statement that she was going to make a diagnosis of gram negative sepsis."

The court asked if Helms was going to testify about gram negative sepsis. I said that Helms was going to testify in rebuttal to Dr. McKinivan and that it was critical. McManus decided that it was too late in the day and adjourned court, putting an end to Helms's testimony. P&G had a right to insist that Helms be recalled the next day for cross-examination, but they agreed to excuse him as a witness rather than have him come back and possibly be allowed to testify on the gram negative sepsis issue. Helms had a busy schedule the next day, after having arranged things in order to testify on such short notice. He asked me if he could be excused and, since I wasn't certain McManus would let him testify on that point anyway, I agreed not to recall him.

I reviewed Helms's limited testimony as I packed my briefcase for the day. There wasn't enough there to counter McKinivan, just the note that Pat had been included in Iowa TSS cases that Helms had compiled.

Closing arguments to the jury were scheduled for the next day, and that would take most of my preparation time that evening. I knew I'd have to spend some of that time contacting Pat's ob-gyn, Dr. Shirk, to see if he could rebut McKinivan—otherwise, all might be lost.

16

"Why didn't Mr. Riley call Dr. Shands to testify? She could have flown up on the same plane with Dr. Dan."

Closing argument of P&G attorney.

After eleven days of listening to testimony from witnesses and looking at hundreds of exhibits, the jury was ready to hear closing arguments. McManus ruled that both sides would have no more than an hour for closing arguments despite my objections that both the fact issues and the legal issues were far too complex for such a limitation. What was worse was that I had to save some of that time for a rebuttal. So it narrowed the hour down to about forty-five minutes for my main argument.

I could not understand how McManus expected me to point out the highlights of sixty-five hours of testimony in such a short time. P&G was happy with the limitation because they didn't need long to create doubt. I was reminded of my Scottish grandfather Kyle's favorite saying about any jackass being able to kick a barn down while it took a carpenter to build one. P&G knew we had the carpenter's role in this case and that proving Pat had TSS and that tampons somehow caused it would be a lot more novel and complicated than building the umpteenth million barn in Iowa, I thought.

McManus didn't think arguments mattered that much, and a lot of lawyers share that view, feeling that the jurors have made up their minds long before it's time to argue. But my experience and post-trial interviews suggest otherwise, and I wanted to make the best argument I could—and an hour just wouldn't be long enough.

So we worked until 2:00 a.m. when, after considering and, in most cases, rejecting, hundreds of bits of evidence and exhibits, I had completed an outline of the message I wanted the jury to take with them to the jury room.

P&G's task was simpler to carry out. Its closing argument had already been shaped by the criticisms and suggestions of the three juries in the secret mock trials. P&G knew what explanation for the company's conduct would appeal to a jury and what attacks on the Kehm evidence would succeed. All P&G's attorney would have to do was to follow the script developed in Lincoln, and if the last mock jury verdict was an accurate barometer, P&G could anticipate victory.

Driving home from the office, I thanked Nan for all the help she had given me in the case. She had attended every court session and had reported on the effect that the evidence seemed to be having on the jury.

"How do you think we're going to do?" I asked.

"We're going to win," she said without hesitation.

"I'd feel better about it if I hadn't left Mrs. Beauregard on—she can't seem to smile enough at P&G's attorneys. Every time she has, I kick myself for going along with Starr."

"You're always a pessimist while the jury is out no matter how well the case went," she countered.

"But I've never left a family friend of an opposing attorney on the jury—that's the sort of dumb thing a law school student is taught not to do. If she hangs the jury or, worse, talks them into a defense verdict, I ought to get out of trial work and draw wills for a living."

"You've said that before and everything has turned out all right."

"But I didn't have the whole town and half the country watching how the case turns out."

After four hours of fitful sleep, Nan and I were on our way back to the federal building. We met Mike, who helped carry the display easel and the large blowups of the P&G memos to the courtroom on the third floor of the building.

I had been right when I said half the country would be listening; local and network reporters had filled the courtroom.

Before closing arguments began, I briefly called Dr. Shirk back to the stand. Pat's ob-gyn specialist challenged the testimony of Dr. McKinivan that Pat had an infection of the uterus. He told the jury the infection was on the cervix and in the canal to the uterus, not the uterus itself.

I rested my rebuttal and could begin the closing arguments.

With a deferential "May it please the court," I turned to the jury:

> "In my opening statement a little over two weeks ago I began by saying on September 2, 1980, Pat Kehm used Rely tampons for the very first time, and just four days later she was dead. She died because Procter & Gamble was more concerned about momentum in the market-place. They were more concerned about the profits from Rely tampons than warning their customers of the possibility of harm, warning them of knowledge that they had."

I then told the jury that I wanted to lay to rest the feeble claim of P&G that its personnel did not know what to say in a warning in the summer of 1980. I showed the jury the blowup of the June 27, 1980, P&G memo to its area managers in which P&G described TSS and its symptoms—the one that instructed them not to initiate discussion about TSS.

Glancing momentarily down the line of P&G attorneys at the counsel table, I looked back at the jury and asked:

> "Did they think we are so dumb out here in Iowa that we can believe that Procter & Gamble, with all of its public

relations people, all of the staff and platoons of lawyers
and note-takers and legal assistants, all of the talent that
$643 million in net after tax profits can buy, that they
couldn't find the talent to write a warning that people
could follow?"

I argued that if P&G had helped spread the word about
TSS instead of keeping quiet, the Mercy Hospital emergency
room physician might have heard about TSS and saved Pat
Kehm's life by proper diagnosis the night before she died:

"If they had done that, Dr. Jacobs has said in effect Mrs.
Kehm would be alive today. And it's as simple as
that . . . all they had to do is say if you get sick, it's not
going to hurt you to remove the tampon and use a napkin . . . on the second of September, two years ago, Pat
Kehm was in good health. She lived, she loved . . . at
one point she asked the nurse, 'Am I going to die?'
". . . and her heart stopped. They tried to resuscitate
her and couldn't. And one of the family, I don't remember now who it was, had to call the mother and say we
lost our baby. That's real people we are talking about.
This is not some statistic somewhere, some file in Procter
& Gamble's office. This was Patricia Kehm."

The facts were overwhelming, I argued, that tampons were
a factor in TSS in menstruating women, pointing to the seven
different epidemiological studies. I referred to the testimony
of the treating physician who tried to save Pat Kehm's life and
contrasted that with a P&G company doctor McKinivan who
"came in as she did in Denver and will in Portland and wher-
ever else they need her."
Holding a box of Rely, I said:

"Look at the box that's in evidence. You won't find anything on there. Certainly not a warning, certainly not
ingredients, nothing but slogans. They spent millions of
dollars to come up with a name Rely, because it's catchy,
but they quibble about spending $70,000 on clinical tests,
$500 to pay a woman to test these tampons."

I referred to the P&G memo that expressed concern about the impact of TSS on P&G but told the jury it would not find any company memos expressing concern over its customers' welfare.

> "And if Mr. Harness, Mr. Fullgraf and all the others, had been concerned, Pat Kehm would be alive and Mike would have his wife that was his childhood sweetheart, and his children would have their mother. It's as simple as that."

Turning to the anticipated P&G attack on Tierno, I asked the jury:

> "If he is a crackpot, why then did Procter & Gamble offer him grants of money even after they say his tests weren't duplicated? You have to have one of two inferences from that. Either he was on the right track, and is knowledgeable and competent, or they wanted to buy his silence."

After arguing that the evidence supported the tampon and TSS connection, I asked the jury to award adequate compensatory damages to the Kehms:

> "Now we are talking about a human life and that's not easy to put in dollars and cents, but I'm going to give some suggestions. The economists testified that the value of those services, based on minimum wages, and you can't buy with minimum wage in most cases, there are exceptions, but you can't buy the kind of attention that a mother gives to a husband and her children. But minimum wage for cook, nurse, teacher, housekeeper, launderess, chauffeur."

After glancing again at the P&G attorneys, I continued:

> "Now there was some ridicule about how many chauffeurs there are in Cedar Rapids. I will tell you how many there are. Every mother is a chauffeur, babysitter, secretary, bookkeeper, and in many cases pays the bills, seamstress, shopper . . . A wife is on call 24 hours a day."

I spoke about the pain and suffering that Pat Kehm had endured:

> "The mental anguish that she went through when she knew or suspected she might die . . . knowing that she was going to leave those two little girls alone."

Referring to the two Kehm children, I told the jury that Mike had not brought the two little girls into court:

> "It was our right. We could have had them sitting there every day, paraded them in every day to prey on your sympathy. I'm not going to do that. I didn't do that. They don't need that additional trauma anyway.
>
> "That little girl in that picture, that little baby is going to wonder what her mother was like. It was so unnecessary. They don't have that mother for one reason, because Procter & Gamble wouldn't spend a penny or two to tell Mrs. Kehm what they knew. That's what it would have cost, a penny or two a package."

I addressed the argument that Pat Kehm is dead so there is nothing that can be done about it.

> "You can't quantify a mother's love and affection and comfort, but that is an element of damage you are entitled to award here. The law says that's the only remedy. We can't bring Mrs. Kehm back, but that's no out for the defendants. They can't say, 'well, you can't bring her back, therefore don't make us pay anything.'"

I reviewed the evidence that showed that P&G knew the risk of TSS with tampons in June 1980 but continued to promote Rely aggressively.

> "They knew that a warning could cause some people to think about whether they would buy Rely and that would hurt them in the marketplace."

I turned to the need for a punitive damage award:

"Mike Kehm brought this lawsuit because they let his wife die. They let the mother of Andrea and Katie die, and the company hasn't learned a thing. They won't admit that Rely tampons are a possible cause. They won't apologize. You know, if they had done that, if they had contacted Mr. Kehm and said we may have been at fault, we are sorry, do you think he would have had the fire that he undoubtedly has and deservedly has?

"I think it's fair to say that the nation is watching what you people do. You have a responsibility for the people of America to set an example. Punitive damages need to be awarded here, not for the Kehms, but for all of us; not to make the Kehms better off, but to make all of us better off—so it won't happen again, so we will send a message to Mr. Harness and all the others.

"I have a daughter who wants to be a lawyer. She pointed something out to me that I think is worth repeating. Rely was only one product, and P&G had many. They wouldn't have missed it. But the Kehms had only one wife and mother."

I thanked the jury for its attention and sat down in my chair at the counsel table. I had spoken for fifty minutes. The young P&G attorney, Warbasse, who had grown up on the farm next to juror Beauregard, had not been assigned any speaking role in the trial. I half expected P&G would call on him to deliver the closing argument. I'd have considered it even more likely if I had known about the P&G mock trials and how the closing argument had taken shape in Lincoln. Instead, P&G assigned the other local lawyer, who had taken an active part in the mock trials, to deliver the prepared argument.

He charged that it was easy to make accusations at a big company like P&G, and to fan the accusations with sympathy, anger and prejudice. And he asked the jury to consider the evidence and not the sympathy in the case. Recalling for the jury the uncontroverted evidence that it was necessary to have all the symptoms of TSS in order for a person to be diagnosed as having TSS, he pointed to the absence in the hospital records of a reference to a rash:

> "You may be very ill and you may have diarrhea, and you may have vomiting, and you may have a fever, but if you don't have rash and you don't have these other things, you don't have toxic shock."

The attorney then referred to the fact that 500 million Rely tampons had been sold between 1974 and 1979 without a problem. Citing the testimony about a wave of staph infections that flooded hospitals in the fifties and then disappeared, he suggested that history was repeating itself—that mutations of staph strain had suddenly appeared. It was something that P&G wasn't responsible for and couldn't anticipate, he claimed. He quoted Schlievert that a small number of people lacked the antitoxin to the TSS staph strain:

> "Dr. Todd and Dr. Schlievert, the world's leading authorities, say they don't have an answer and an answer probably isn't going to be here for years. We are operating in a medical and scientific vacuum."

He reminded the jury that Rely went off the market in 1980 and there had been more TSS cases in Iowa in 1981 than the year previously. Then, noting that I had witnesses flown in from Atlanta and New York at a cost of thousands of dollars a day, he asked why the emergency room physician, Dr. Ziblich, wasn't called when he was only four blocks away. And why a third doctor by the name of Haupt wasn't called as a witness.

> "And isn't it kind of interesting that Mr. Riley didn't bring Dr. Haupt here? You know, he is an anesthesiologist here in Cedar Rapids. It wouldn't have cost too much money to bring him up here. But he isn't matching up with toxic shock, apparently, so that is why you folks aren't going to get to see him."

After using one hand to praise the doctors for "valiantly trying to save this woman's life," he used the other to criticize them and try to create more doubt:

> "But they threw away the most important piece of evidence, the tampon. If we would have had that tampon saved, there would be no discussion as to what kind of tampon or brand it was. There would be no discussion or speculation as to whether or not it contained any bacteria. But we don't have that. And it is kind of hard to defend yourself when the main piece of evidence has been thrown away. Because, again, we weren't there. We were back in Cincinnati."

Referring to the conversation between Jacobs and me on September 29, 1980, and the doctor's memo and notation that "we did not talk about the IUD," the attorney commented:

> "I'll bet there are a lot of things he didn't talk about. The weather, the Iowa football team. There were a lot of things. But he put that in voluntarily. He was still thinking IUD."

Returning to the theme of doubt and uncertainty, the attorney told the jury:

> "And now Dr. Jacobs and Dr. Quetsch come in here and they say it was caused by Rely tampons and that caused her death. But have they told you exactly how it was caused? No. They don't know. If they don't know then how can they say that? I don't know. Maybe you folks can figure that one out."

On the subject of the tampon's role, the P&G attorney said sarcastically that only Tierno claimed to have an explanation.

> "You remember Tierno, his wife said, 'Philip, there is a strange disease called Toxic Shock Syndrome. You are bright. Why don't you go down to that laboratory in New York and find the answer.' You know what Philip did?

He went down there and in thirty days he found that answer, an answer that eluded the scientists of the world."

Referring to the charges that Tierno had made for a deposition he gave to P&G in another TSS case, the attorney told the jury:

"And doesn't it make sense, and again dwelling on your common sense, doesn't it make a little sense that it is kind of peculiar that the scientific community isn't breaking down this man's door and they are not bombarding him if he has the answer. Maybe they just think he is some kind of nut. Some kind of a nut charging $5,000 for a deposition and $1,200 to read it. But you know, folks, maybe he isn't such a nut. Maybe we are all missing the boat if we could get a job like that."

He asked the jury where the scientific proof was that tampons cause TSS:

"We brought the leading authorities here. Todd, Schlievert, Feinstein, Evans. They say there are any number of possible causes but they don't know the answer. I ask you to contrast those people with Dr. Dan who is a hundred percent sure of everything right now but isn't it important and interesting he didn't disagree with his boss, Kathryn Shands, or the FDA in the summer of 1980 who all reported that there was no proof of causal relationship?"

The P&G attorney turned to the question of whether Rely had been adequately tested for safety. He claimed that Rely had been extensively tested, not just in P&G's own labs, but at places like the Mayo Clinic, Wayne State University and Baylor College of Medicine:

"And if Mr. Riley thinks we can buy off the Mayo Clinic and the Baylor College of Medicine in Houston, then he must think we really have a lot of money and he must think that these people are really some people down there."

He recalled the testimony of former FDA Commissioner Ley, who said that P&G's kind of testing was so conclusive and exact and exhaustive that it was the same as would be required of a prescription drug.

The P&G attorney justified his client's failure to warn in the summer of 1980 by reminding the jury that Dr. Shands had told Hassing on August 21 that she was going to continue to use tampons and that she saw no need for a warning.

I winced at the reference to the Shands matter, which I had been helpless to rebut. The P&G attorney then held out the withdrawal of Rely as a humanitarian act that cost P&G millions of dollars:

> "Not because we thought they were dangerous but we were in a controversy and we didn't have the answers and we were uncertain."

He then pointed to a blowup of a letter from Shands that commended P&G for "voluntarily withdrawing Rely and for financing a large advertising campaign to warn of the association of TSS with Rely tampons."

Despite the P&G attorney's knowledge that Shands could not testify, he asked why we had not called the CDC official to the stand, why she had not "flown up on the same plane with Dr. Dan."

Preparing to return to the counsel table, the P&G attorney closed by saying: "We leave our 145 years reputation for honesty and safe family products in your hands and await your decision."

My mind raced through the many points I would like to make in the six hundred seconds left for rebuttal. I felt I should answer the questions about the rash and the failure to call Dr. Ziblich, the emergency room physician who saw Pat Kehm the night before she died. As my eyes moved from juror to juror, I told them that Mike had seen the rash and that Dr. Quetsch had seen it also; that Dr. Helms, who had testified without any fee, said that he had missed a rash in a TSS case due to a tan the victim had and that it wasn't uncommon to miss it.

As to Ziblich, I called P&G's accusation about his not testifying a phony issue and an act of desperation. I pointed out that P&G had taken the depositions of all other doctors and the nurses and they could have taken Ziblich if they had wanted to do so. They could have called him as a witness if he had anything to offer beyond what was in the hospital record. I told the jury the case would have taken another week if all persons having any connection with the case were called as witnesses. I said that Ziblich was a typical M.D. in 1980 who didn't know about TSS because knowledgeable firms, like P&G, did nothing to help spread the alarm.

I turned to the P&G claim of extensive testing of Rely. I said that even if the testing had been adequate prior to June 1980, it became immaterial after the CDC study showing a significant association with TSS and that P&G should have warned. As for Tierno, if he was a crackpot:

> "Why did they want to meet with him the Saturday before this trial was to begin? Why did they offer him those grants that have come into evidence, and he wouldn't accept them? The one honest man."

As for P&G excusing itself from responsibility for the misdiagnosis of Pat Kehm at Mercy Hospital the night before she died because P&G was "back in Cincinnati":

> "They did everything they could, and you read those memorandums, they did everything they could to see that the information didn't get out:
> "'Don't initiate the discussion.' Then they want to say, 'we were back in Cincinnati, it wasn't our fault.'"

As to the Shands letter commending P&G, I reminded the jury of Dan's testimony that the CDC was trying to be diplomatic—they were dealing with a large company and needed their cooperation. Then I challenged P&G's argument that I could have brought Shands to Cedar Rapids to testify if she had had anything to say that would have helped his case:

"All those P&G attorneys know the government doesn't let CDC officials testify in these proceedings."

The P&G attorney objected but McManus merely noted that I had one minute of time left.

So I repeated that P&G knew Shands couldn't testify and that P&G was stooping low when it tried to blame Mercy Hospital for not recognizing TSS when P&G tried to keep the doctors from knowing about the disease.

I concluded by telling the jury that the attorneys in the case would go on to other trials but that this was the Kehms' only case—their only opportunity to be fairly compensated and the only opportunity for society to be redressed by punishing P&G's kind of conduct.

It was 11:30 a.m. on Tuesday, April 20, 1982, when I had returned to my chair at the counsel table, and all that remained was for McManus to read the instructions of law before the jury retired to decide whether Rely tampons killed Pat Kehm.

PART
FIVE

The
Verdict

17

"We would like to get the first portion if not all of the jury instructions . . . we have come to rather a stand-still."

Jury request to Judge McManus.

After first peering over his reading glasses to ensure that he had the jury's attention, McManus glanced downward at the papers in front of him, and began to read aloud. He told the jury the time had come to instruct them as to the law governing the case. He warned them to follow the law regardless of any opinions they might have as to what the law should be. He added:

> "The law does not permit jurors to be governed by sympathy, prejudice or public opinion."

He explained that the burden of proof was on the Kehms but that absolute certainty wasn't necessary. The proof had to be supported by the "preponderance of the evidence," which McManus said means to prove that something is more likely so than not so. He said the issue was whether Rely tampons were defective and that the law considered a product defective if a warning should have been given and wasn't.

He instructed the jury that a manufacturer doesn't guarantee that no harm will come from using the product. All the manufacturer is required to do, he said, is to make a product that is free from defective and unreasonably dangerous conditions, pointing out that "unreasonably dangerous" meant a defect in the product that would be unreasonably dangerous to the user in the normal or foreseeable use.

He told the jury that if Rely tampons were defective and Pat Kehm died as a result, the jury should award compensatory damages for the support and services that she would have contributed to her husband and children had she lived, for the children's loss of their mother's companionship, affection and guidance. He said the jury could also award damages for pain and suffering she sustained after the onset of her illness and until her death, plus the $7,446.04 for her medical, hospital and funeral expense.

McManus instructed the jury that it could award punitive damages if it found that in the summer of 1980 acts or omissions of Procter & Gamble showed a "heedless and utter disregard" for the rights of Pat Kehm. He explained that the purpose of punitive damages was not only to punish the wrongdoer but to serve as an example or warning to others not to engage in such conduct. McManus concluded by telling the jury that its verdict must be unanimous. Everyone rose as the jury was escorted out of our courtroom.

After the jury had left, P&G's attorneys obtained McManus's permission to remain in the courtroom to await the verdict. They were grandstanding in the hope that the jury would see them when they were taken out for meals and would be impressed with their continued presence after the trial.

After lunch with Nan, Michele and Dean Rotbart, the *Wall Street Journal* reporter who had written the Bergdoll stories, I tried to get some work done on other cases. At 4:30 p.m., the receptionist said the federal clerk was calling, and I raced to a phone only to learn that there was not a verdict—the judge wanted the lawyers to come to his chambers to discuss a request from the jury. At the federal building, McManus gave the P&G attorneys and myself a photocopy of a note from the jury that requested a copy of "Gray's Medical Dictionary, if possible, or any other medical dictionary." It was signed by Dean M. Helgins, jury foreman.

I smiled since there was no dictionary known as Gray's. I figured that someone on the jury remembered my reference in closing argument to *Gray's Anatomy*. I had mentioned it in connection with the location of the staph infection—whether it was in the canal to the uterus, as Pat's doctors said, or in the uterus proper as P&G's McKinivan claimed. But I was concerned by the jury's need to see a medical book. This meant that one or more jurors was troubled by McKinivan's claims about the site of the infection. If the jury was looking that closely at the medical evidence, then they must have doubt that Pat had TSS and they might never get to the question of the defect of the tampon.

"I'm not inclined to give the jury a medical dictionary," McManus told us. "What do you gentlemen have to say about it?" he asked.

In a rare act of agreement, P&G's attorneys and I concurred that it would be inviting error to give the jury a technical manual and let them be misled or confused in the attempt to interpret and apply medical definitions. McManus adjourned the meeting by advising us that he would tell the jury it may not have a medical dictionary but to continue its deliberations.

At 6:06 p.m., the jury sent another note to the judge. The note McManus handed us this time read:

> "We would like to get the first portion if not all of the jury instructions, due to confusion on instruction breakdown, we have come to rather a stand-still. Jury foreman Dean M. Helgins."

The first part of the instructions dealt with the question of liability and not damages. That meant the jury was having trouble agreeing among themselves that P&G was at fault. McManus told us that he didn't like juries to have the written instructions in the jury room, but in this instance, he would let them have a complete set of instructions.

I was not in a good mood when I got home. The jury's request for a medical dictionary and the portion of the instructions dealing with liability enhanced my usual pessimism. I sensed a verdict for P&G was in the offing and that I had failed Mike and his two little girls. Nan reminded me that I was always pessimistic and usually wrong, but it didn't help my state of mind.

Tired from a long trial and lack of sleep the night before, I went to bed shortly after 9:00 p.m., the hour that the jury was to be sent home for the night if they hadn't reached a verdict. The next morning, Mike called asking what was happening. I told him it wasn't unusual for the jury to stay out this long. I suggested he might consider hanging around the courthouse like the P&G attorneys were doing.

> "I doubt there's a psychological benefit but it would be even better for a grieving husband to be waiting for the verdict than for a bunch of highly paid attorneys."

I dropped by later in the morning and found out that there was no chance of the jury seeing either Mike or the P&G attorneys, so I told Mike to forget it and go home and wait for my call.

The call came after lunch. The Deputy Clerk of Court was on the line. He told me that the jury had returned a verdict in favor of the Kehms and against P&G. I was instantly pulled out of my depression. They had awarded $300,000 in compensatory damages, he said. This was the highest verdict in Iowa's history for the death of a housewife, and after the misgivings I had during jury deliberations, I was relieved that the jury found Rely was responsible for Pat Kehm's death. My elation subsided when the clerk said the jury had not awarded punitive damages. Because of the Hassing testimony about Shands and the warning, I wasn't shocked that the jury let P&G off the hook on punitive damages. But I felt that even if it was only one dollar, P&G deserved to have a punitive damage award against them—just to tell the world that their conduct was reprehensible. Hassing had saved P&G from that fate.

Mike shared my relief at winning as well as my disappointment that P&G had escaped punitive damages. I suggested that he come to the law firm so we could meet the press together. I reminded him that the important thing was that we had won. We would not give P&G the satisfaction of seeing us downcast about the failure to win punitive damages.

When we met the assembled reporters, I told them that P&G had put the entire weight of the corporation's resources into the case, hoping to win and setting a precedent in the hundreds of other TSS cases pending against the company. "Procter gambled," I said, "and lost." When a reporter informed me that P&G was claiming a victory because the verdict was substantially less than what we had originally sued for and because there were no punitive damages awarded, I asked if P&G was planning to appeal the case. I followed up the point:

> "Seems to me that if they had won the case, they sure as hell wouldn't be thinking of appealing. Only losers appeal. If P&G thinks it won the case, I'll expect a check tomorrow for $345,000. I bet I don't see one for a long time."

One of the reporters broke in:

> "I thought the verdict was $300,000."
> "That's right, but we have a law in Iowa that allows interest from the time a suit is filed and as of today, we've earned $45,000 in interest on the $300,000."

Later in the day, the claim of a moral victory by P&G gave way to the new P&G claim that the verdict was based on sympathy rather than the evidence. When that report was published, a juror, who requested not to be identified (but who I learned was Mrs. Beauregard), snorted and told a reporter that it was sympathy for P&G that kept the verdict down and excluded punitive damages.

Both our office and P&G attorneys interviewed the jurors. To our mutual surprise, my biggest supporter had been Mrs. Beauregard—the most vociferous proponent of a punitive damage award against P&G. The banker's wife and the secretary, probably from their association with the side of management, had trouble believing that a big corporation could do anything wrong. It took some urging by the other six jurors to convince them to find against P&G for compensatory damages. From the interviews, we learned that the jury was hesitant to start a precedent by awarding punitive damages. They were aware that P&G faced several hundred other TSS suits. As one juror put it, P&G would be bankrupt if it were fined for punitive damages in every TSS case—a fate the jury felt would be undeserved since the CDC's Dr. Shands had said a warning wasn't necessary, and in addition, P&G had already lost many millions as a result of Rely being taken off the market.

P&G did file a motion for a new trial and, when McManus turned it down, appealed to the Eighth Circuit Court of Appeals, which finally heard oral arguments at the University of Nebraska Law School on February 17, 1983, nearly a year later.

P&G general counsel McHenry later told me that the company appealed because it was the first time in its 145-year history that a P&G product had been found responsible for a customer's death. I felt there was a less sentimental reason. A decision by the Eighth Circuit Court of Appeals upholding the Kehm verdict would make it easier to TSS victims to prove their cases. It would make P&G more willing to settle TSS claims for fair sums. P&G had been capitalizing on the economic disadvantage to TSS victims of waging litigation war with the company. Claims worth $50,000 were settled for $10,000 or $15,000 by some victims because it would have cost them $50,000 to prove the case against P&G.

That is what it had cost Mike Kehm. Experts who left the comfort of their homes in Atlanta or New Jersey to travel to a small midwestern city understandably expected to be compensated at a much higher rate than what they would charge for consultations in their own back yards. Even the price of local experts did not come cheap. Dr. Jacobs, the family practitioner who had tried to save Pat Kehm's life, submitted a bill for $3,000 for the time he spent in the witness box.

When the trial had ended and even before the expense of an appeal, Mike Kehm had paid out about $7,000 of his own money for out-of-pocket expenses of litigation and owed about $45,000 more. If the verdict would be upheld, Mike would have enough money to pay the expenses, but the expert witnesses and other creditors were not expecting to wait a year or two to be paid. Moreover, if the verdict would be set aside, Mike would face bankruptcy. I proposed a solution.

After the Kehm verdict had been reported in the national news media, I had been deluged with requests for help from lawyers for TSS victims all over the country. I'd spent many hours on the phone answering questions of TSS lawyers who had yet done little investigation into the subject. I had learned that James Brien of Mayfield, Kentucky, had ordered a transcript of the Kehm trial from the court reporting firm that had provided P&G with its "dailies." The court reporters had charged Brien $3,100 for the transcript, based on the official rate of $1.05 a page. I arranged to make a copy of Brien's transcript and then offered it for $750, or one-fourth the price, to lawyers who had contacted me for advice on their TSS cases. I also offered copies of all plaintiff's exhibits, including the P&G documents obtained in the search in Cincinnati, plus legal briefs, pleadings and the like for the sum of $450.00.

I told Mike what I planned and explained that all of the proceeds received from the sale of the transcript and the documents package would go to Mike's bills for the trial. Neither the firm nor I would be reimbursed for our efforts in copying or forwarding the materials. The only expense that would be deducted from the receipts would be postage and actual costs of photocopying, most of which was done by outside photo-copy firms. Mike gratefully gave his approval to the plan, which would help him as well as other TSS victims.

Because the cause of TSS was still scientifically unproven, and the Kehm case was the only one that had resulted in a judgment against a tampon manufacturer, my offer generated considerable interest from plaintiffs' lawyers. More than seventy lawyers ordered materials from the Kehm case, including such well-known personal injury firms as Melvin Belli's of San Francisco, Gerry Spence's of Jackson, Wyoming, and F. Lee Bailey's of New York. By the time the last dollar had been recorded, Mike had been reimbursed in full for checks he had already written and expenses he had paid or still owed when the trial ended. At the same time, TSS victims obtained the information that had been acquired on Mike Kehm's behalf at

Now, TSS victims were gaining the evidence that strengthened their hand in negotiations with P&G. The lawyers ordering the transcripts could be allowed to read Dan and Tierno's testimony into the record in their cases and would not have the expense of the expert witness fees. P&G was furious. They waited for me to make a mistake. And I did.

It was my intention to include in the documents package only exhibits that had been admitted into evidence during the Kehm case in open court. Inadvertently, some P&G documents, which had not been offered into evidence, were sent out. They had been marked as exhibits but withheld because they were repetitious of others that were offered. A communication problem with Michele was the cause. I told her to send "plaintiff's exhibits"—meaning those offered into evidence at trial. Michele thought all documents were "plaintiff's exhibits" if they had a sticker to that effect whether offered or not. I should have been more specific.

Many of the nonoffered exhibits had been obtained under the protective order that I had unsuccessfully resisted and that McManus had required as a condition for inspecting P&G's records. Attorneys for P&G learned in early August 1982 that

I was furnishing documents on the exhibit list to TSS lawyers. Yet, P&G let two months go by before attempting to protect the supposedly valuable trade secrets. On October 4, 1982, P&G filed an application to have me cited for contempt of court for violating the protective order by disclosing P&G documents to third parties.

Before filing the application, P&G attorneys had leaked their intention to do so to the Cedar Rapids news media. This led to a local radio station quoting an anonymous lawyer as describing the practice of "selling evidence" as legal but "sleazy." Paul Harvey repeated the story on his nationally syndicated noon news show. When the local radio station and Harvey learned that the courts favor unfettered exchange of evidence between lawyers and that all the money went to Mike's benefit, both issued "on the air" retractions and apologies.

I called Calder in Cincinnati when I learned of P&G's threat to file contempt charges. I advised the P&G attorney that some documents had been sent out that had not been admitted into evidence but that none of them appeared to have any trade secret value as they all related to Rely tampons and not other P&G products that were on the market. I had notified the lawyers receiving the documents that some had not been admitted into evidence and should be treated confidentially. I asked Calder if there was any reasonable solution for the problem short of a contempt hearing. Calder said that he couldn't speak for P&G but that it would be his recommendation that there be no contempt application if I recalled all of the documents pending a ruling by McManus on an application that I had filed with the federal court to release all P&G documents from the protective order. I said that sounded reasonable and to let me know if P&G agreed to Calder's recommendation.

Three days later, October 4, 1982, Calder told my son, Peter, that P&G would only forego the filing of a contempt application if, in addition to retrieving all of the documents and refunding the money collected for Mike Kehm, I withdraw the application to release all P&G documents from the protective order. I had filed the application for two reasons—

one, so that I could continue to pay off Mike's debt by making the court documents readily available to other attorneys and, also, to release other documents that I had obtained from P&G that were never on the exhibit list. They wanted me to sell Mike's rights down the river in order to avoid a contempt charge.

The contempt application was filed when I refused P&G's terms. In April 1983 the federal courthouse in Cedar Rapids became the scene of another trial. This time it involved P&G's claim that valuable trade secrets had been disclosed in violation of the protective order. At the trial, P&G narrowed its claim to the contention that only two of the documents sent out contained trade secret material. One of the documents dealt with the production schedule for a proposed deodorant Rely tampon, which was never marketed, and the other with a non-deodorant Rely tampon. I could not conceive of how either contained any value to a competitor, particularly in view of the fact that Rely tampons had been off the market for nearly three years and no objective person could claim Rely tampons would ever have marketability in the future. P&G attorneys claimed to have logged $40,000 in legal fees prosecuting the contempt action before the start of the four day contempt trial had even begun. They asked that the court award P&G at least that amount against me.

McManus held that the violation of the protective order by me had not been willful but that there was a violation nonetheless. He awarded P&G $10,000 in attorneys' fees, or one-fourth of its claim. P&G attorneys conceded privately that the company's costs in prosecuting the contempt action exceeded a quarter of a million dollars.

It would not be until December 1983, more than three years after Pat Kehm's death, that the court would reject P&G's appeal of the Kehm verdict, and the corporate giant would be finally forced to pay the judgment owing to the Kehm family, which, because of accumulated interest, came to $404,000. When Mike came to pick up the check for his share of the proceeds, I had more to give him than money. Since the trial had ended, I had obtained some information to share with him about P&G's behind the scenes handling of the TSS crisis—information that I felt he would find just as disturbing as I had.

18

"From the FDA pragmatic viewpoint, TSS is <u>not</u> an important disease. . . . They <u>do</u> recognize the public relations aspects."

P&G memo regarding
the company's meeting with the FDA,
November 12, 1980.

In the summer of 1982, while the Kehm case was on appeal, Shands left the CDC to take a position at Emory University in Atlanta. When I learned of this in December 1982, I wrote to her about Hassing's claim—that Shands told him in August 1980 that she saw no reason to warn tampon users about TSS. Now that she was free of CDC restrictions, I asked Shands to give me a deposition to set the record straight—and to put a stop to Hassing's repeating that claim in other TSS cases around the country. A few days later, she called me from Atlanta.

Shands said she was already aware of Hassing's testimony in the Kehm case, and it was obvious as she spoke about it that she was still angry about it. She then confided that Hassing and another P&G official had contacted her in Atlanta as soon as she left the CDC. They told the former CDC toxic shock

257

expert that they had come "to offer P&G's help in shielding
her from harassment by plaintiffs' lawyers in TSS litigation."
Shands made it clear to me that she resented P&G's solici-
tousness, which she knew masked its real concern that she
would make herself available to victims in TSS litigation.

She had pointedly reminded Hassing that she did not make
the statement he was attributing to her and she expected Hassing to stop making the allegation. During the meeting in Atlanta, Hassing told Shands that P&G would be interested in
funding her in whatever job or research that interested her,
and he implied that she would be "set for life" if she accepted
their offer.

Armed with this information, I filed Requests for Admissions in a new TSS case I was handling against P&G. In them,
I asked P&G to admit the facts that Shands had related to me.
Shortly after filing the Requests, I was contacted by Nick
Patton, a lawyer for a Texarkana, Arkansas, TSS victim. Patton told me he was preparing to take Hassing's deposition, and
I informed him of Hassing's testimony in the Kehm case about
the alleged Shands statement and Shands's denial of it. Patton
promised to find out what Hassing would say now that Shands
was available as a witness to contradict him.

At the deposition Patton took on June 23, 1983, he asked
Hassing:

> "Did Dr. Shands tell you at a meeting in the summer of
> 1980 that she saw no need for a warning nor a withdrawal
> from the market of the product?"
>
> "We never really discussed either of those points that I
> recall," Hassing conceded.
>
> "You testified in Iowa that she made such a statement
> did you not?" Patton then asked.
>
> "I don't believe so," Hassing replied.

Thus, Hassing not only recanted on the claim that the top
TSS investigator of the CDC saw no need for a warning, but
he claimed not to recall making the statement in the Kehm
case.

Aware of his visit to Shands in Atlanta, Patton first asked the P&G scientist why he and another P&G official had traveled from Cincinnati, Ohio, to Atlanta, Georgia, to see Shands. Hassing said it was to "find out what she was going to be doing careerwise." Patton then asked:

"Did you go to Atlanta especially to see Dr. Shands?"
"Yes."
"And solely for the purpose of being able to keep up with where she was?"
"Yes."
"I don't understand the necessity if all you were interested in Dr. Shands was where she was going to be, to have two men going to Atlanta, Georgia, to find that out. It seems to me that a simple telephone call could do that."

Hassing replied:

"Well, we concluded collectively it was just going to be better and I guess more complete to be able to just have a face to face conversation and that was certainly not the first time we had all been to Atlanta. So, we just decided to go down."

The deposition I wanted Shands to give never took place. The ex-CDC official was cool to the idea of formal participation in any court proceeding. She had offered to write a letter to me "setting the record straight." I told her that would not be admissible as evidence and I'd need her deposition, which could then be used in all court cases. I mentioned I was going to be in Atlanta in December 1982 to watch the Iowa football team play in the Peach Bowl and suggested this would be an ideal time for me to take her deposition. This wouldn't work out, Shands told me, since she was going to be in the Caribbean over the Christmas holidays. She did promise to call me after the first of the year to discuss a deposition further. She never called back, but I realized I had what I needed to contradict Hassing—the knowledge that the P&G scientist had contacted Shands after the Kehm case, his explanation for it and Shands's angry response. And, after I filed Requests for Admissions in the new Rely TSS case, P&G knew I knew and Hassing had no choice but to recant when he was next under oath—at the Patton deposition.

In the summer of 1980, P&G had remained silent and let people die. It then engaged in questionable conduct in the defense of TSS litigation, including the suppression of scientific discovery. But, I told Mike, as bad as P&G has been, it is not the only guilty tampon company. Tampax resisted putting a TSS warning on its boxes of tampons until the law required it, more than two and a half years after tampons were first linked to TSS. A Tampax fact sheet inside the box allayed women's fears about TSS by boldly stating: "Tampons do not cause Toxic Shock Syndrome." While acknowledging in smaller type that some studies showed an association between tampon use and Toxic Shock Syndrome, the Tampax fact sheet pointed out that the illness was believed to be caused by a bacterium known a *Staphylococcus aureus*. Yet, Tampax's own market research showed that many women who were asked to read the Tampax fact sheet were lead to believe that they were safe from TSS if they used Tampax and that only Rely tampons were involved with TSS.

Tampax even threatened at one point to sue the American College of Obstetricians and Gynecologists when it learned that the respected group of medical specialists planned to issue a warning against the use of superabsorbent tampons in the fall of 1980. To their credit, the doctors went ahead with their warning, although it had no apparent influence on the FDA or the tampon companies.

Canada's equivalent of the FDA required TSS warnings on tampon boxes by December 1980, but it was not until two years later that the FDA required such a warning for tampons sold in this country. Tampax had complied with the Canadian requirement on a warning for all boxes sold in that country but did not do so in the United States until the FDA finally required it. In joint defense of the FDA and Tampax, Dr. Clayton Thomas, Tampax's medical director, made an intriguing observation during a deposition in a TSS case. Denver lawyer Kaufman, who was at that time representing a Tampax TSS victim, questioned Thomas about why Tampax warned Canadian customers but not those in the United States:

"Let me ask you this; do you have any evidence to believe Canadian women are any different than American women?"

"Every woman is different from every other woman. I know there are literally a great number of differences with respect to ethnicity, with respect to climate, with respect to the average number of children born to each mother, the average income, the socio-economic level is different in the two countries, the crowding is different. So that I cannot say I have knowledge that they are, either. I have a lot of knowledge that they can be quite different."

"The warning was put on the box in Canada but not in the United States?"

"That is my understanding, yes, sir."

"Is that because Canadian women are viewed by Tampax, Incorporated, as being more important than American women?"

"No, sir."

In the course of further research following the Kehm verdict, I found out that Congress passed the Medical Devices Amendments to the Food, Drug and Cosmetic Act in 1976. Three classifications of medical devices were established by the FDA. Tampons are classified as class II medical devices, as are about 60 percent of all medical devices. But the FDA had not promulgated performance standards for any of the classes.

Congressman John D. Dingell and Victor Jaffra of the FDA discussed tampons, toxic shock and performance standards at a hearing on July 16, 1982:

DINGELL: "Tampons are class II devices, are they not?"

JAFFRA: "Yes, sir."

DINGELL: "Now that means they were placed in class II because the FDA believed that a performance standard was essential to make the device safe for use, does it not?"

JAFFRA: "That is one of the conclusions that justify placing a device in class II, yes, sir."

DINGELL: "But there is no performance standard with regard to that?"

JAFFRA: "There is none."

DINGELL: "That is approximately six years after the 1976 law. It is how long after the discovery of the relationship of tampons with Toxic Shock Syndrome?"

JAFFRA: "I think in the fall of 1980 we had enough statistical information to infer that the TSS and tampons were related."

The FDA's conduct in the summer of 1980 was as shameful, if not more so, than that of the tampon industry. It should surprise no one when private corporations act in what they think is their own best interest. But the interest that the FDA is obliged to advance is the welfare of the public. The FDA did not seem to realize that, at least in the summer of 1980. Its solicitude seemed to be for the tampon industry rather than the consumer. The only statement on TSS issued by the FDA was the July *Drug Bulletin* and that had been written and sent only at the prodding of the CDC task force on TSS.

Many women's lives might have been saved had the FDA conducted a vigorous campaign to warn American women about TSS in the summer of 1980. Instead, Lillian Yin of the Bureau of Medical Devices of the FDA told P&G's Gordon Hassing that the CDC had "jumped the gun" regarding the association of tampon usage with TSS. According to a P&G memo, she expressed surprise that the tampon manufacturers had not objected more vigorously to the CDC about the validity of CDC I and the Wisconsin study. The FDA seemed to resent the Centers for Disease Control's intrusion into their jurisdiction over tampons. On August 21, 1980, Jerri B. Perkins, M.D., of the FDA Office of Health Affairs, wrote to Lillian Yin that the CDC study and other public health studies were only:

> "Preliminary and suggestive of a relationship between TSS and tampon use. In view of this, I believe it was premature for the FDA drug bulletin to have made recommendations."

In three weeks, the CDC II would be released and the FDA's hand would be forced. The FDA did not consider TSS worthy of its time during the summer of 1980. As P&G official E. R. Wilson was to note in an interoffice memorandum of a meeting with the FDA and Procter & Gamble held on November 12, 1980:

> "From the FDA pragmatic view point, TSS is *not* an important disease. . . . They *do* recognize the public relations aspects. It is their understanding that CDC is trying to elevate TSS to a reportable disease."

The lack of cooperation between the FDA and the CDC reached a point where FDA commissioner Goyan wrote CDC director William H. Foege, M.D., on July 16, 1980, requesting FDA participation in a design of a prospective study of TSS since "tampons are regulated by FDA." Perhaps the FDA's attitude toward the consumer was best summed up by the statement of Lillian Yin, who, in a telephone conversation of July 9, 1980, had asked P&G's Gordon Hassing to put ingredient labeling of tampons on the boxes if the cost was "minimal." That way, she said: "We're both off the hook, even though the consumer activists won't learn anything and no one will read it."

The academic and scientific communities did not cover themselves with glory in the TSS story, either. With the exception of Tierno and his colleague at NYU, Bruce Hanna, TSS researchers gratefully accepted and in most instances eagerly sought the huge tampon companies' research grants. The recipients included scientists who had been in the forefront of

TSS research, like Todd and Davis. The latter two, coincidentally after receiving the grants, both published articles that were sympathetic or helpful to their tampon company sponsors. Galask, from Iowa, who had told me in early October of 1980 that tampons undoubtedly played a role in Toxic Shock Syndrome in menstruating women, would later join the P&G stable of defense witnesses in TSS litigation.

But, the conduct of Bergdoll of Wisconsin and Schlievert of Minnesota raises the most questions. Both collected a number of tampon company research grants. Bergdoll, in his state-owned laboratories at the University of Wisconsin, discovered as early as 1981 that *Staph aureus* toxin production was greatly increased in the presence of all tampons. In the case of Rely, he found toxin production was increased twenty to a hundredfold over other tampons. However, the results of those tests had not yet been published by him when the December 1983 issue of the *Journal of the American Medical Association* took Bergdoll and Procter & Gamble to task for possible suppression of his scientific data.

Bergdoll denied that he could be improperly influenced by tampon company funding of his work. However, when Bergdoll became aware of P&G's displeasure with a press release in which Bergdoll took the tampon and TSS connection for granted, he immediately wrote the company a letter expressing his "humble apologies" if it caused P&G any embarrassment. A Bergdoll press release subsequent to his "humble apologies" letter to P&G, questioned the connection by referring to his test on the role that tampons play in TSS, "if indeed, they play a part."

In denying that the tampon company grants in excess of a half million dollars weighed in his decision not to publish his 1981 toxin production tests, Bergdoll claimed that the tests were "only preliminary." P&G used his claim in refusing to furnish the test results to TSS victims. Yet, in 1985, Bergdoll submitted the supposedly "preliminary" 1981 data to a scientific journal for publication. Even after doing that, he resisted a new court action to release his data and he continued to

claim, through his attorneys, that the findings were only preliminary.

Why did Bergdoll submit an article on the data for publication? The answer may be found in the article itself. Bergdoll
had long chafed at the criticism of the *Journal of the American
Medical Association* and others for his failure to release his data.
When he finally decided to quiet criticism by submitting an
article to *JAMA*, he wrote it in such a negative manner that it
begged rejection. In addition, it didn't measure up to the usually high scholarly writing standards of Bergdoll's scientific
contributions, as if Bergdoll didn't care if it were accepted for
publication, which it wasn't. Thus, Bergdoll was in the unusual position of being able to take satisfaction in being rejected
since it allowed him to reassert his claim that his data on toxin
production were not worthy of publication.

The University of Wisconsin lent its prestige and resources
to the Procter & Gamble campaign to keep the Bergdoll studies
secret. It furnished lawyers and even enlisted the Wisconsin
attorney general's office to fight attempts by TSS victims to
depose Bergdoll or obtain the data implicating Rely. The university claimed "interference with academic freedom in research" as a basis for moving to quash a subpoena for Bergdoll.
For three years, Bergdoll continued to claim his toxin production tests were only preliminary and the university argued that
requiring Bergdoll to tell the results of his research would
"inevitably tend to check the ardor and fearlessness of scholars,
qualities that are so fragile and so indispensable for fruitful
academic labor." United States district court judge Meredith
of Missouri accepted this argument and denied a St. Louis
TSS victim's husband and child the Bergdoll data. P&G then
settled with the family, thereby avoiding a review and possible
reversal of Meredith's decision by the Eighth Circuit Court of
Appeals. P&G then used the Meredith decision as a precedent
to persuade other courts to keep the Bergdoll data from TSS
victims' hands.

What the University of Wisconsin did not point out to the
court was that virtually all of Bergdoll's research work at the

University of Wisconsin, whether TSS related or not, was done for private corporations. Since the 1940s, food corporations have supported the Food Research Institute of the University of Wisconsin. Bergdoll was the first employee of the institute when it began in 1946 at the University of Chicago, and Bergdoll has dedicated his life to it. Over the past two decades, no food corporation had contributed larger grants to the Institute than Procter & Gamble.

And the University of Wisconsin benefits greatly from private corporation funding. It takes 43 percent of each grant for general university purposes unless the corporation makes an outright "gift" for the research project—one with no strings attached.

In tampon research, P&G has refused the outright "gift" approach and has insisted on such restrictions as the right to review manuscripts before they are submitted for publication—even though it has to pay 75 percent more to fund the research than if it made an outright gift.

The successful suppression of Bergdoll's findings did a disservice to the reputation of the University of Wisconsin, not only because victims of TSS were denied the evidence that would have helped them obtain justice but, more tragically, because the most harmful tampons for sale after Rely had been recalled, those with the superabsorbency component polyacrylate, remained on the market until as late as 1985. The majority of the TSS deaths after the recall of Rely involved those highly absorbent tampons advertised by their manufacturers, Tampax and Playtex, as "Super Plus" tampons. Those two tampon manufacturers recalled their Super Plus tampons in the spring of 1985 after they learned of the pending release of a scientific study by a Harvard group that strongly implicated polyacrylates and one of Rely's components, polyester, in toxin production. A $10 million dollar punitive damage award in Wichita, Kansas, against Playtex in a Super Plus TSS case might have also played a role in Playtex's decision.

Had the Bergdoll findings been publicized in 1981, would not the tampon companies have been forced to remove all tampons containing synthetics, or at least those causing the higher levels of toxin production? Since Bergdoll was funded by tampon companies, as was the Harvard group, the tampon companies could not easily dismiss their sponsored findings as biased or flawed. Moreover, had the tampon companies ignored published findings by Bergdoll, they would have exposed themselves to the potential for astronomical verdicts for punitive damages. It is one thing to play down unpublished data which the researcher himself labels as "only preliminary." It's quite another to ignore published data from a scientist of Bergdoll's stature—especially one who had received the kind of confidence in his ability that several hundred thousand dollars of funding represents. The release of the Bergdoll findings might have forced tampon manufacturers to return to the relatively safe, all cotton tampons, and an indeterminate number of women's lives would have been saved. I personally am aware of five cases of women who died of TSS in 1982 while using tampons with synthetic components.

Bergdoll followed his 1981 laboratory tests with an equally interesting experiment in 1983. Suspecting that cotton might have special properties to explain the fact that TSS did not surface until the fifth decade of tampon usage (when synthetics replaced cotton in tampons), Bergdoll devised a new test. Using the same type of syringe he had used in his earlier experiments to measure toxin production, he placed cotton, blood and 20 micrograms of toxin inside the syringe. After a short interval, he squeezed the cotton with the syringe plunger to force the fluid out. Unlike the earlier experiments, when bacteria were present to produce toxin in the syringe, Bergdoll knew that there could not be any more than the 20 micrograms of toxin that would be squeezed out of the syringe. However, since 20 micrograms went in, 20 micrograms should have come out. To Bergdoll's satisfaction, his hunch had proved right. No toxin came out. The cotton, apparently, would not release it.

Of course, a syringe is not a vagina, a point Bergdoll would emphasize in justifying his refusal to release this evidence that damages P&G's contention in Rely litigation that recent incidents of TSS had nothing to do with the change in tampons from cotton to synthetics. But Bergdoll's test offers a laboratory explanation as to why Dr. Haas's original all-cotton Tampax did not cause TSS. Even if a toxin was produced as a result of an environment created by the cotton tampon (which is debatable), any toxin would apparently be retained by the cotton and not pass through the vaginal wall into the woman's body where it would cause illness.

Procter & Gamble claims the decision not to publish or release his experiments and findings was Bergdoll's. But P&G had been promptly furnished with all of Bergdoll's findings under the terms of the funding that it provided Bergdoll, and P&G then resisted court efforts by Rely victims of TSS to see either Bergdoll's or the company's test results. P&G had the obvious motive of keeping TSS victims from using the test documents to overcome P&G's defense that no scientific evidence of a tampon and TSS connection existed.

While Bergdoll's silence furthered P&G's goal of keeping damaging evidence from seeing the light of day, Schlievert helped the tampon companies by devising a dubious test of tampons and *Staph aureus* toxin.

After the Kehm trial, Schlievert had sent P&G's attorney Woodside a bill for his witness fees and expenses of $1,401.72. In a letter accompanying the bill, he expressed disappointment in the Kehm verdict, wished Woodside luck in the future and offered "to help with future cases in any way I can." That unusual promise of help was soon forthcoming. With a grant from Kimberly-Clark, manufacturer of the Kotex brand of tampons, Schlievert conducted a laboratory test designed, it seemed, to prove that tampons inhibit the production of a TSS toxin, what I would sarcastically come to call his "tampons are good for you test." *Obstetrics and Gynecology* rejected an article based on his results because the testing was flawed.

Schlievert had failed to use blood as a medium, although one need not be a scientist to know that that fluid is present in the vagina during menstruation. He knew the CDC had shown

that certain leachables from tampons can inhibit toxin production but that the leaching effect is negated by simply adding
blood to the culture medium. One might wonder whether
Schlievert wanted the effect negated. Moreover, Schlievert shook
the flask containing the tampon components and the *Staph aureus* at two hundred revolutions per minute. This introduces
oxygen into the culture medium and causes maximum toxin
production, whether or not tampons are present. But it is an
unrealistic test since it doesn't duplicate the virtually oxygen-
free environment of the vagina. By aerating the flask to achieve
maximum toxin production without tampons present, Schlievert
had designed a test that would inevitably show toxin production was not increased in the presence of the tampon. When
you reach the limit, you can't exceed it, and that's all that
Schlievert's test showed. Moreover, because tampons, when
added to the culture medium, reduce the capacity of the medium to be fully aerated, there was a slight reduction in toxin
production, leading tampon companies to point to Schlievert's
test as proof that tampons do not play a role in TSS. *Obstetrics
and Gynecology* would not publish the manuscript in its original
form. He resubmitted the article with substantial changes, and
it was eventually published.

Although Schlievert obtained his reputation in TSS research circles for his published article describing the isolation
of Exotoxin C, I learned he wasn't the actual discoverer. It had
been Dan and Shands from the CDC who pointed out the
toxin to Schlievert. They had visited Schlievert at UCLA to
look over his data claiming a toxin, Exotoxin A, was responsible for TSS. Dan and Shands saw what should have been
obvious to Schlievert, that while Exotoxin A was found in the
strain of *Staph aureus* implicated in TSS, it was also found in
about 95 percent of all other strains of *Staph aureus*. Schlievert's
data also showed that Exotoxin C was present in all *Staph aureus*
cultures from TSS victims, but it was produced by only 5
percent of all *Staph aureus* strains.

Dan and Shands argued vigorously with Schlievert to get
him to understand his own data. Schlievert did not agree at

first and submitted a manuscript to the *Journal of Infectious Disease* in which he contended that Exotoxin A was the TSS toxin. The manuscript was rejected, and at that time, he turned to Dan and Shands and asked them to rewrite the manuscript to make it worthwhile to publish. Schlievert didn't even want to review what they wrote. "Don't even send it back," Schlievert told Dan and Shands, "I trust your judgment."

The two CDC doctors, overwhelmed by their own work loads, reluctantly acceded to Schlievert's request. Despite the fact that their rewrite of the article substituted their thesis about Exotoxin C for Schlievert's Exotoxin A, they graciously submitted the article for publication with Schlievert's name as the lead author, thereby establishing Schlievert's reputation in TSS research as a discoverer of the TSS toxin.

Except for Dan, Shands and the editors at the *Journal of Infectious Disease*, no one knew about Schlievert's identifying the wrong toxin—until a TSS trial in San Jose, California, in December 1982. Schlievert was called as an expert witness by Johnson & Johnson, the manufacturers of o.b. tampons.

While delighted to have a chance to finally refute Tierno, Schlievert lost his composure when the plaintiffs' lawyer handed him the rejected manuscript in which he had claimed that Exotoxin A was the responsible agent for TSS. Schlievert thought the rejection of his manuscript was a closely guarded secret. His credibility as a witness in the o.b. case was destroyed as he asked in an agitated voice where the attorney got the manuscript, pointing out that he hadn't "released it to people." Once again, the result was a jury verdict that endorsed Tierno's views and rejected Schlievert's.

The CDC is one of the few heroes in the TSS story. However, the CDC cannot escape some criticism for its role in the needless deaths from Toxic Shock Syndrome in 1980. Although well-meaning, CDC investigators not only thought like scientists but they spoke like scientists. The result was a semantics problem that gave moral support to the tampon industry and lulled many tampon users into a false sense of security.

Specifically, the CDC investigators used the simple word "cause" in its technical sense. On too many occasions, CDC task force members would emphasize that tampons do not "cause" TSS. They would say this when interviewed by news media, when answering letters from inquiring doctors and laymen and at general briefings. In doing so, they were being technically correct. They would point out—as the *MMWR* of June 27, 1980, did—that tampon use "by itself" does not cause TSS. The CDC meant that tampons, acting alone, would not cause TSS but, under the right conditions, could do so. P&G and the other tampon companies knew what the CDC meant, but the lay public was confused by it.

In the summer of 1980, the American public needed understandable information—not scientific hair-splitting. It would have been far more helpful if the CDC had simply stated the fact that tampons were capable of causing TSS sickness and death in some menstruating women. The CDC should have explained that certain bacteria in the vagina and a lack of immunity to the toxin were also necessary but that all women were at risk since it wasn't known who had the bacteria present and who was immune. Had the CDC taken that position instead of speaking in scientific parlance, there would have been less confusion or misunderstanding on the public's part.

How would one expect the typical teenager to comprehend Shands's statement that "TSS is not caused by tampons, but is merely associated with them." And as a group, teenagers were most susceptible to TSS.

Shands, as director of the CDC task force on TSS, was somewhat naive in dealing with P&G. She treated P&G scientists as colleagues to whom the usual scientific courtesies should be extended and reciprocated, when, in fact, they were adversaries. She was unaware of the objectives of P&G to manipulate her and Dan, as set forth in the October 17, 1980, memo from P&G's Geoffrey Place. This memo, which I had shown to Dan at our first meeting, outlined a "fundamental strategy" of convincing the two CDC doctors that P&G could "enhance their ability to be seen as leaders of the crusade against TSS." Place had proposed a visit to the CDC to convince the task force of developing "a close working relationship between P&G and CDC." As a result of P&G's contact with Shands, she supplied them with an advance copy of the January 30, 1981, *MMWR*, which covered the TSS story in the United States from January 1970 through December 1980.

A memorandum by P&G's E. R. Wilson discusses his telephone conversation with Shands of January 27, 1981, following her trip to Cincinnati:

> "Dr. Shands assured me that we would find a new version of the MMWR more palatable than the original version."

Shands was not corrupt. She was simply too trusting.

An irony about P&G's decision to remain silent in the summer of 1980 is that it ultimately cost the company its tampon product. The decision, in August 1980, to delay a proposed warning because it was "premature" was based on P&G's fear that such a warning might hurt the momentum that Rely had had in the marketplace. In hindsight, had P&G issued a warning soon after it learned about CDC I and used its sophisticated advertising and marketing skills to educate the public, Rely might still be on the market and P&G would be making millions from it. Granted, there would have been a temporary reduction in tampon usage, but this effect would have cut across the board, and Tampax, as the market leader, would have suffered the greatest loss in sales. The great majority of women can safely use Rely and other synthetic tampons. With proper education on TSS in the summer of 1980, the incidence of the disease could have dropped significantly, and early removal of the tampon at the first symptoms of TSS would have resulted in mild cases that would not have met the CDC reporting requirements. Death from TSS might have been virtually nonexistent. CDC II would not have been necessary, and Rely would not have been singled out for the criticism that CDC II inevitably brought.

But P&G hoped to weather the storm, and it "positioned itself as part of the tampon pack" in order not to lose even one percentage point in market share. The other tampon companies didn't warn either, but there is some poetic justice in Procter & Gamble's product being banned since it had launched the superabsorbency race that led to the TSS epidemic of 1980. There may be a final lesson in the TSS story. The inaction of the FDA in the summer of 1980 and its foot-dragging in requiring TSS warnings on tampon boxes demonstrates once again that the American consumer cannot depend solely upon its government to promote product safety. The TSS story shows the role the private lawsuit can play in product safety. A financial lesson lasts the longest. Lawsuits filed by Mike Kehm and the other victims of TSS made a financial impression on Procter & Gamble. The speed with which P&G recalled the Duncan Hines products with the pesticide EDB in 1984 may be proof that the giant household products company has learned something from having been sued for the damage done by Rely tampons.

And the Kehm case helped victims of other product defects. From the beginning, Mike pursued the litigation against P&G in the hope that teaching the company a lesson would help other people. I was reminded of that when an attorney for the manufacturer of the Dalkon Shield IUD told me about a court case he had lost in Minneapolis.

The IUD manufacturer, A. H. Robins Company, had objected to the introduction of CDC studies showing an association between the Dalkon Shield and pelvic inflammatory disease in women. Robins's attorney made the same argument that P&G had made against admitting CDC I and II into evidence. The judge trying the IUD case said he agreed with the manufacturer's argument yet he had no choice but to admit the studies in view of the decision by the Eighth Circuit Court of Appeals in the Kehm case.

Epilogue

Although the special design and composition of Rely made it the most dangerous tampon, its removal from the market did not end tampon-induced TSS. The extent to which it reduced the incidence of illness and death among American women is debatable since many Rely users simply turned to other superabsorbent tampons.

Ironically, at the very hour the Kehm jury returned its verdict on April 20, 1982, a twenty-four-year-old housewife and mother, Tammy Ann Farris, died of Toxic Shock Syndrome in Enid, Oklahoma. She was using Playtex Super Plus tampons, a brand that would be withdrawn by Playtex in 1985. Mrs. Farris may have shared the belief of many tampon users that only Rely caused TSS.

Toxic shock cases continue to be reported to the CDC but in a haphazard manner. In 1984, there were 461 reported cases. Of the approximately 80 percent that were menstrually-related, 99 percent were using tampons at the time of their illness. Dr. Margaret Oxtoby of the CDC speculated in March 1985 that the CDC statistics are conservative estimates because, in her opinion, doctors are diagnosing and treating the disease but not reporting it. Since doctors are not required to report TSS cases, Dr. Oxtoby believes they are no longer taking the trouble of "calling the CDC and filling out a number of forms," now that there is little publicity about the disease.

The removal of Rely, earlier diagnosis and improved treatment appears to have lowered the death rate from tampon-related TSS. Based upon the assumed underreporting of TSS to the CDC and the known mortality rate of TSS, it is estimated that at least 12 women died from TSS in 1984 compared to 42 in 1980. Another 368 tampon users had close brushes with death. The tampon companies seem to accept these deaths and illnesses as the cost that they and a relatively small number of their consumers have to bear—the unlucky consumers with their lives or health and the companies with a small percentage of their profits going to settle claims. It's just part of the cost of doing business—like advertising or shipping costs.

The attitude of the tampon companies was summed up by Edwin Shutt, Jr., president of Tampax (now Tambrands), who was quoted in the *New York Times* on March 4, 1985: "We had a flurry of ads in the fourth quarter of 1980, after Rely was withdrawn, listing what the symptoms are, but as any good advertiser would, we went back to selling the benefits of the product." In truth, Tampax's attitude in the fall of 1980 was to continue business as usual. A Tampax interoffice memo of December 12, 1980, recommended against TSS warnings and concludes that Tampax should "permit the education of the consumer to remain in the hands of competitors." When Tampax did warn about TSS in the fall of 1980, it did so by pointing the finger at Rely—which was no longer on the market. And Tampax was the last to print a TSS warning on the box when the FDA finally required it, more than two and a half years after the first CDC study linking TSS to tampons. They still don't have a warning on boxes sold in England since the government doesn't require it.

Long before the death of Mrs. Farris, Playtex knew of laboratory tests showing Playtex Super Plus ranked high in causing the production of TSS toxin. In addition, Playtex officials learned in 1981 of the epidemiological study known as the Tri-State Study, which showed that superabsorbent tampons, including Playtex Super Plus, increased a woman's chances of getting TSS many times over the less absorbent tampons.

While males and nonmenstruating females can get TSS from wounds or other infection sites in the body, such cases constitute only about 20 percent of the total TSS cases, and there is little or nothing that can be done to prevent such infections. Menstrually-related TSS, on the other hand, is preventable. The prevention lies with the elimination of superabsorbent tampons and the return to the all-cotton tampon.

If the FDA were to act in the public interest, it would approve only tampons made of cotton and ban the use of carboxymethylcellulose, polyester, polyacrylates and other synthetics in tampons. Synthetics that do not enhance toxin production may exist or are capable of being developed. Before allowing any such new synthetics in tampons, there must be comprehensive testing, first in the laboratory and then, only if the laboratory tests are favorable, under carefully controlled monitoring of volunteers who are informed of the risks and the tell-tale signs of TSS—unlike the millions of women who were unknowing guinea pigs for tampon testing of Rely and the other superabsorbent tampons.

Although the manufacturers have removed some of the highly absorbent materials from tampons, there is nothing to stop their reintroduction. In fact, Tampax began using carboxymethylcellulose (CMC) in 1985 in its Super Plus tampon. CMC and polyester were the two superabsorbent synthetics in Rely tampons.

Tampax's decision to use CMC was based upon a Tampax-financed laboratory study by a Harvard group headed by Edward Kass, M.D., a specialist in infectious disease. Kass had testified for Tampax as an expert witness in TSS litigation. Tampax reportedly funded Kass's research group with the bulk of the $4 million that it has spent on TSS research.

Kass released the results of his study on June 5, 1985, and implied that his group had solved the problem of tampons and Toxic Shock Syndrome. The study implicated polyester and polyacrylate as the villains, concluding that the amount of toxin provided in the laboratory tests varied with the level of magnesium present and that both synthetics caused the level of magnesium to be optimal for toxin production.

Most of the news media did not read the fine print in the Kass report, and the result was newspaper headlines and reports on radio and television that the toxic shock puzzle was solved. It hasn't been.

Knowing about the Kass report in advance, Tampax had quietly withdrawn polyacrylate from its Super Plus tampons in February of 1985, and Playtex, the only other manufacturer using polyacrylates in its tampons, followed suit the following month. Since Rely was the only tampon that had contained polyester, Kass told the Associated Press that current tampons were safe. At least one newspaper, the *Washington Post*, noted an anomaly. Kass's study, which *Time* magazine called "the magnesium connection," exonerated synthetics such as carboxymethylcellulose and viscose rayon while indicting polyester and polyacrylates. Yet, many TSS victims, including both those who survived and those who didn't, used tampons containing CMC or viscose rayon but not containing polyester or polyacrylates. Kass conceded to the *Post* that his study did not explain those TSS cases.

Kass's study was published in the June 1985 issue of the *Journal of Infectious Disease*, a reputable scientific journal that Kass served as chief editor for a number of years. A close look at the fine print in the Kass article reveals three interesting statements. First, Kass concedes that his laboratory experiments, like the one Schlievert devised under a grant from Kimberly-Clark, "were conducted in the absence of blood," an astonishing deviation from the actual menstrual environment. Next, Kass concedes that since it can be expected that blood and menstrual fluid may vary in the amount of magnesium ions available to the synthetic fibers, "future experiments will need to take this variation into account." Lastly, Kass admits that what happens in the laboratory may not be relevant *in vivo* (i.e., in the body).

I contacted Tierno and Dan separately after the release of the Kass report. Tierno told me he felt the Kass study was flawed, and Dan, who is now a senior editor of the *Journal of the American Medical Association*, agreed. Both scientists commented on the credibility problem of a scientific study so heavily funded by a private corporation with a substantial investment interest in the outcome. Neither thought that such a report as flawed as the Kass study would have been published by the *Journal of Infectious Disease* had Kass lacked his prestige and influence as a former chief editor of the journal.

Even Schlievert disagrees with the Kass conclusions. The June 6, 1985, edition of the *Minneapolis Star-Tribune*, in the same story that reported on the Kass study, quoted Schlievert as saying that "it is very premature to say that magnesium is associated with TSS." But such views were either ignored or not sought in the national media's rush to announce the good news.

Substantial damage to public health has been done by the widespread publicity given the Kass report and the failure of the news media to get a second opinion. The erroneous impression has been created that tampons are safe, now that none contain polyester or polyacrylates. But women will continue to get sick and some will die from the tampons that contain synthetics other than polyester and polyacrylates. And, having been lulled into a false sense of security about the safety of present-day tampons, it is not inconceivable that the death toll will be even higher because women may delay treatment thinking they have the flu. That's what happened to thirty-four-year-old Judy Hutsell of Kansas City, Missouri, who was using a Tampax brand that contained neither polyester or polyacrylates when she contracted TSS and died in July of 1982. Mrs. Hutsell delayed treatment because she thought she had the flu, apparently in the belief that Rely was the only tampon that caused Toxic Shock Syndrome. The misconception created by the Kass group that tampons are now safe is likely to create more Judy Hutsell scenarios.

The burden on the FDA to take action in the public interest is even greater now as a result of the widespread publicity given the Kass report. If the FDA lacks the will to ban synthetics, it should at least require a continued educational campaign about tampons and TSS by the tampon manufacturers. Although two years late in the making, the current FDA regulation on a TSS warning falls far short of what is needed. It only requires a message either on the box or on an insert that reads:

> "Attention: Tampons are associated with Toxic Shock Syndrome (TSS). TSS is a rare but serious disease. It may cause death. Read and save the enclosed information."

There are several faults with such a message. First, it isn't likely to be read. If the consumer already has heard about TSS in the past and thinks that she knows what there is to know about it, as Playtex's own studies of consumer awareness reveal, then there is no motivation for her to read the message. To attract the reader's attention to the message about TSS and tampons, the warning should declare: "Warning. This tampon can kill you. Read this, it may save your life."

Such a warning is necessary because many women (55 percent in one Playtex consumer awareness study) believe that the TSS problem is related only to Rely tampons. Moreover, most women in that Playtex study assumed that the tampon manufacturers would make the products safe after the TSS epidemic of 1980.

They were not alone. Trained specialists as well assumed the best about tampon manufacturers. More than a year after the 1980 tampon and TSS epidemic, a Playtex awareness study of obstetricians and gynecologists revealed that less than 10 percent of those doctors believed that any of the tampon brands still on the market were made with superabsorbents!

Another problem with the current warnings is that they don't correct the erroneous belief of many women that if they used a particular tampon in the past without getting TSS, they are safe if they continue to use that brand of tampon. An appropriate warning would explain that past safe usage is no assurance of future avoidance of TSS, pointing out that changes often occur in the kinds of bacteria present in the vagina and that if a particular strain of *Staphylococcus aureus* should appear, the use of the tampon could induce the bacteria to produce the deadly toxin.

Tampon manufacturers sell their products by advertising on television and radio as well as in the newspapers and magazines. They do not sell them by the messages they put on the boxes—if they did, they could save a lot of the money they spend in advertising. They know the way to influence the consumer to buy is through the advertising mode. The companies should be required to employ the same mode to educate women about TSS, especially young women who constitute the age group most susceptible to the disease. The FDA should require the tampon manufacturers to spend a certain amount of their advertising dollars on a TSS educational campaign, using television and the other media. This campaign must not be a one-shot transaction like the one that briefly followed Procter & Gamble's forced removal of Rely from the market. Since a new group of women reach puberty every day, the advertising campaign must continue as long as tampons cause Toxic Shock Syndrome. Such a campaign will help prevent tampon users from being lulled into a false sense of security by prior safe use of the tampons, from forgetting a message heard about TSS a long time before, or from the false assurances of the Kass report.

In my opinion, there are several reasons why the FDA has not taken meaningful steps at this writing to protect American women who use tampons. For one thing, the pressure is off the FDA because the number of potential TSS victims is relatively small. While this is true, medical science does not know which tampon users will get TSS. Every menstruating woman using tampons is at theoretical risk of dying from Toxic Shock Syndrome. Without regular monthly testing of a woman's vaginal flora, she cannot be assured that she is safe from TSS. A special blood analysis can show whether the woman may have developed antibodies to the TSS toxin, but it has not been established what constitutes a safe level of antibody.

The early misconception that TSS had been eliminated by the recall of Rely tampons took the pressure off the FDA to act. The Kass report may have the same effect. The few deaths annually are apparently acceptable to those same people in the FDA who told P&G at one time that they did not consider TSS a very important disease. They may even feel that if the TSS victim fails to read or understand the information about TSS on the box or in the package insert, it is just too bad and that the consumer assumes whatever risk there is.

Another reason the FDA may not have acted at the time of this writing is because important scientific evidence about synthetics and cotton has been withheld from the public—a direct result of the fact that P&G is still defending TSS cases and has no reason to see that data such as Bergdoll's is available to TSS victims who are suing P&G. Thus, it is not only past TSS victims who have suffered from court-imposed sanctions against release of P&G's sponsored research, but the general public suffers whenever important health information is withheld.

I obtained the Bergdoll materials as a result of an enlightened decision by a woman judge in Kansas—a decision P&G appealed unsuccessfully to the Kansas Supreme Court. But a condition of my obtaining the Bergdoll test documents limits my use of them to cases where I represent a victim. I cannot otherwise publicly distribute them.

Procter & Gamble and the other tampon manufacturers have not been under any court order barring public distribution. They, in fact, provided the funds for the studies, despite Bergdoll's and P&G's claim that Bergdoll "owns the studies." But, it is not in the tampon companies' interest to do so as long as they have TSS cases to defend. Nor is it in the interest of the manufacturers of synthetic tampons still on the market, all of whom have millions of dollars in revenue at stake. The only synthetic-free tampon available at this time is a Tampax product called "Original Regular." Tampax's other three styles contain synthetic components.

Federal budgetary restraints limit the CDC's list of priorities and, with it, truly independent research into TSS. In fact, the CDC was reduced to pleading for funding from the tampon manufacturers to carry on its TSS research—a plea that fell on deaf ears because of the CDC requirement that there be no strings attached to any such funding.

The bottom line on Toxic Shock Syndrome is that women will continue to die painful and terrorizing deaths from the tampon-induced disease because of the combination of FDA apathy and corporate self-interest. Unlike deaths from some dread diseases, these TSS deaths are preventable. All it would take is voluntary action by the tampon companies to return to an all-cotton tampon, or action by the FDA requiring the companies do so.

In addition to warning unsuspecting women about tampons and TSS, as well as encouraging action to eliminate synthetics from tampons, Mike Kehm and I hope this book will serve another purpose: to change governmental attitudes, so that the next time a study by the Centers for Disease Control, or some other reputable agency, suggests a product may be responsible for illness or death, our government will give the public, and not the product, the benefit of the doubt.

A Note from the Author

Many of the events of Pat Kehm's life and death recounted here are based on my interviews with her family, friends, doctors and the hospital personnel who attended her in the emergency room. I have attempted to recreate some of my conversations with them in order to give the reader an idea of who Pat was and of the circumstances that led to her early death from Toxic Shock Syndrome.

Other conversations quoted in the text occurred throughout the discovery stage of the lawsuit against Procter & Gamble, including those with expert witnesses for both sides. Additionally, Bruce Dan, formerly of the Centers for Disease Control, provided the material relating to CDC I and II. Attorneys for other TSS victims and their families, and survivors of toxic shock, further fleshed out the narrative. Many of their statements disclosed here are from my best recollection; others have been transcribed from extensive notes or tapes made during our discussions.

In most instances, quoted material set off from the text has been taken from interrogatories, depositions and documents marked for exhibit during trial. All trial testimony has been transcribed verbatim from court transcripts. Many of the quoted documents are from P&G's files and include interoffice memos on Rely and TSS, P&G meetings with the Centers for Disease Control and the Food and Drug Administration, letters to P&G-funded scientists, letters from the funded scientists and communications regarding P&G customer relations and publicity.

Source material for the scientific information on TSS and tampon use is derived from scholarly journals and scores of newspaper articles from the onset of the TSS epidemic in 1980 until this book went to press. FDA publications, records and documents were also reviewed in preparing the text, as were the *Morbidity and Mortality Weekly Reports* on TSS, published by the Centers for Disease Control.

Much of the information about Tampax (now Tambrands) and International Playtex and their roles in tampon-induced TSS was obtained during preparation for other lawsuits I filed on behalf of TSS victims. I am indebted to attorneys of other TSS victims who, both before and after the trial of the Kehm case, supplied material information that they had uncovered about the conduct of tampon manufacturers. Mark Hutton of Wichita, Kansas; Vic Bergman of Kansas City, Missouri; Mike Liles of Fort Worth, Texas; Steve Kaufman of Denver, Colorado; Nick Patton of Texarkana, Arkansas; Bill Travis of St. Louis, Missouri; and Jim Brien of Mayfield, Kentucky, were particularly helpful in this respect.

I am also indebted to my wife, Nan, our daughter, Pam, as well as Amy Pastan, of Adler and Adler, for their invaluable help in editing this book; and, of course, my agent, Nat Sobel, who believed in this book from the beginning.

Index

A

American College of Obstetricians and Gynecologists, 260
American Journal of the Medical Sciences, 227
Annals of Internal Medicine, 142
Askren, Michele, 78, 105–6, 217

B

Bailey, F. Lee, 252
Beauregard, Betty (juror), 153–54, 218, 249–50
Becker, Todd, 77–78
Belli, Melvin, 252
Bennett, John (CDC), 52
Bergdoll, Merlin, 71–72, 113–15, 264–68, 282
Brayman-Lipson, Judy (consumer activist), 37
Brien, James, 251
Buc, Nancy (FDA lawyer), 53, 54, 55, 56, 58, 117–18

C

Calder, Tom (P & G attorney), 138, 142, 143, 152, 209, 212, 215, 253
Cannon, Martin (P & G official), 32, 219
Carlson, John (reporter), 220
Carrigan, Judge James, 74
Carter, Owen (P & G official), 47, 51, 218–19
Cedar Rapids Gazette, 168–69
Centers for Disease Control (CDC): briefings with FDA and tampon manufacturers, 48–49; criticism of CDC I sample size by FDA, 84–85; criticism of handling of TSS investigation by, 270–72; and early reports on TSS, 20–21, 27–28; Epidemic Intelligence Service of, 43; methodology and validity of studies attacked by P & G, 75–76, 129–30, 137, 161, 162–64, 216–18; relationship of publicity to TSS

H

Haas, Dr. Earl E., 81–83, 193
Hahn, Max, 193
Hanna, Bruce, 184, 263
Harness, Edward (P & G chairman), 57–58, 222–24
Harvey, Mary, 75
Harvey, Paul, 253
Hassing, Gordon (P & G product safety), 46, 47, 48–49, 102, 134, 207–10, 211–13, 258–59, 262, 263
Haverstadt, Dale (P & G official), 51
Health Industry Manufacturers Association, 59, 215
Health Research Group (Nader), 84, 85
Helgins, Dean M. (jury foreman), 247
Helms, Dr. Charles, 115, 225–28, 239
Hile, Paul (FDA), 53–54, 58
Hirchma, Kurt (FDA), 38
Hodges, [Federal magistrate] James, 88, 91, 103, 104, 114, 138
Horowitz, Ralph, 75
Hutsell, Judy (TSS victim), 279
Hutton, Mark, 167

I

Imboden, Linda (TSS victim), 65, 102

J

Jacobs, Dr. John: attacked by P & G defense, 154–55, 237; testimony of, 168–73; treatment of Pat Kehm by, 9, 13, 15–16, 21; verifies TSS diagnosis of Pat Kehm, 19–20
Jaffra, Victor (FDA), 261–62
Johns-Manville Company, 67

Johnson & Johnson, 83, 139, 270
Jones, Colleen (Pat Kehm's sister), 5–6, 7, 14, 40, 188–92
Journal of Infectious Disease, 270, 278, 279
Journal of the American Medical Association, 265
Journal of the Nebraska Medical Society, 111

K

Kass, Dr. Edward, 277–79, 282
Kaufman, Steve, 84, 85, 88–89, 91, 92–93, 101, 127, 128, 139–40, 142
Kehm, Andrea, 3–4, 5, 7, 8, 190, 192, 234
Kehm, Katie, 3–4, 5, 6, 7, 190, 192, 234
Kehm, Mike, 89–90, 218; advised on image by psychologist, 152; correspondence with Todd, 132–33; costs of trial to, 251; deposed by P & G attorneys, 80, 81; marriage to Pat, 189; meets with attending physician, 15–16; on punitive damages, 201–2; refuses P & G settlement offer, 138–39; retains Riley, 16–17, 19, 20; testimony of, 195–202; and wife's illness and death, 7–8, 13–14
Kehm, Pat: annual value of services as housewife and mother, 193–94; cause of death of, 160, 161, 169–72, 224–25, 227; family life and marriage of, 4–5, 189–92; illness and death of, 7–14, 195–97
Kennedy, Sen. Ted, 164
Kidneigh, Jon, 85–86, 88–89, 91, 92–93, 101, 127, 128, 139–40, 142
Kreckler, Roland, 168–69
Kuzzler, Doris (P & G), 110–11

ABOUT THE MAKING OF THIS
BOOK

The text of *The Price of a Life* was
set in Janson by Harper Graphics
of Waldorf, Maryland. The book
was printed and bound by
Fairfield Graphics of Fairfield,
Pennsylvania. The typography
and binding were designed by
Tom Suzuki of Falls Church,
Virginia.